Tough Choices

Tough Choices

Health Care Decisions
and the Faith Community

Graydon F. Snyder

Foreword by Donald E. Miller

BRETHREN PRESS
Elgin, Illinois

Tough Choices: Health Care Decisions and the Faith Community

Copyright © 1988 by Graydon F. Snyder

BRETHREN PRESS, 1451 Dundee Avenue, Elgin, IL 60120

*This publication is made possible
through a generous grant from the
Brethren Health Foundation*

Grateful Acknowledgement is made to KCTS, channel 9, Seattle, Washington for permission to quote material from *Hard Choices,* a documentary series on health care ethics; and to Oxford University Press, New York, New York for permission to quote from *Principles of Biomedical Ethics* (1983) by Tom Beauchamp and James Childress.

Library of Congress Cataloging-in-Publication Data

Snyder, Graydon F.
    Tough choices: health care decisions and the faith
community / Graydon F. Snyder.
       p.   cm.
    Bibliography: p.
    ISBN 0-87178-558-7
    1. Medical ethics. 2. Christian ethics. 3. Health—Religious
aspects—Christianity. I. Title.
    R725.56.S69 1988
174' .2—dc 19
Manufactured in the United States of America

To the happy memory of
Dr. D. L. and Martha Horning,
and to the staff of
Bethany Hospital, Chicago, Illinois

Table of Contents

Foreword

Graydon Snyder's book comes at a time when the blessings of modern medicine are accompanied by an unprecedented tangle of ethical problems. Medicine has always been confronted with dilemmas such as how much pain to inflict in the course of a remedy, the outcome of which is uncertain. Medicine has also always worked in situations where human need exceeds technical resources so that choices must be made about who is to receive help and who is not.

From its beginning, medicine has developed on the edge of the sacred and the forbidden. The human body has traditionally been revered, and experiments that are basic to advancing medical science have long been suspect. Western medicine developed in the context of a series of moral and religious judgements, and it is not surprising that the practice of medicine and religion in some cultures are combined in the role of the medicine man or woman. The advances of modern technology and secular science are remarkable, yet the practice of medicine cannot be finally separated from its moral and religious setting.

Though medicine has historically faced moral and religious decisions, such decisions have taken on a new poignancy and urgency in the latter part of the twentieth century. If Western civilization had come to the opinion that, except for quaint sectarian objections to certain treatments, medicine had achieved a moral neutrality and objectivity, more recent medical advances have shattered that opinion. Now it is clearly recognized that moral and religious questions abound on all sides of health care issues.

While the problem of pain has been changed by modern anesthesia, new decisions must be made about when someone has died. Heart and lung machines can sustain bodily functions long after the higher capacities of the brain are lost. The problem of limited resources is compounded by the very fact that medicine can transplant human organs when such organs are in great demand and short supply. If experimentation on the human body in the past bordered on the religious, then research with human genetics and reproduction seems to be tampering with the most basic creative processes of the universe. The moral and religious questions related to medicine have not subsided. On the contrary, they have enlarged.

The moral and religious setting of medicine is not limited to scientists, physicians, and other health care providers. Almost everyone has faced or will face questions about when life has come to an end, or whether to allow further experimentation. Nearly everyone is affected by policies about how many public resources should be spent on health maintenance and who should be helped.

The present book is directed to this very personal side of modern medicine. Snyder is aware that the moral and religious roots of medical decision making place such decisions within the faith community. He is particularly concerned about the Free Church family of churches. This tradition has always been concerned with healing, birth, and death. Yet the whole church, even in an era of morally neutral medicine, has continued to visit and pray for the sick. Snyder shows that the church today is called to an awareness of the moral and religious questions related to health and illness.

Most congregations, in the face of complex new problems related to illness, are ill-prepared to give assistance. Snyder's study is intended to educate local churches so that they may be genuinely caring and helpful. He encourages congregations to develop representative groups that can give support and informed counsel to persons at a time when critical decisions must be made. The idea of congregational health care committees that help work through the moral and religious complexities of health decisions is analogous to ethical decision groups that hospitals are beginning to accept as normal practice.

Snyder is foremost a Biblical scholar. His ideas on death and resurrection are particularly insightful. The book is most helpful, however, in clarifying the religious assumptions of moral decisions related to health and illness. He begins by tracing commonly accepted moral perspectives on health issues and then proceeds to give an alternative biblical and theological stance on these same issues.

Ethicists regularly distinguish between an ethic of rules and an ethic of consequences. For example, the question about telling a patient the truth about dying may be answered much differently by rule ethics than an ethic of consequences. Snyder reviews these traditional ethical stances and then suggests that the church decides on the basis of virtue or narrative. The Bible has both rules and awareness of consequence, but its more fundamental idiom is story telling, that is, narrative. The church lives out a narrative about the love of God that gives context and direction to decisions about health and dying. It becomes clear that the church has a special and important role in such decisions.

Consider four fundamental principles of medical ethics: autonomy, nonmalfeasance, beneficence, and justice. The principle of autonomy protects the right of the patient to decide. This is obvious in the case of the illness of a child, but is also true for an adult.

The principle of nonmalfeasance suggests that the health care provider not leave a person with greater injury than was originally present. Snyder recasts this principle into an argument for the sanctity of creation. The principle of beneficence requires that the medical treatment benefit the patient in some way. Again Snyder shows that a narrative approach reinterprets the situation in terms of God's promise and fulfillment. The principle of justice usually balances the costs and benefits of medical resources. Snyder calls for a *Shalom* approach that looks to the wholeness of life. In each instance he offers a Christian narrative alternative to a secular stance.

The book abounds with insight on important issues. Abortion should be considered in the context of a community covenant, particularly the parental wish for a child, rather than basing a decision on biological conception alone. Death is more than cessation of biological function; it is separation within the community. Distribution of limited medical resources should not favor the wealthy and influential. Therefore, Snyder favors a lottery approach. Genetic engineering does not necessarily violate the divine creation so long as it is responsibly done for human benefit. Christians are to be concerned about life style issues such as drug and alcohol abuse as well as environmental health issues like hunger, pollution, and AIDS. Snyder thus shows the dramatic and far reaching implication of a Christian stance toward issues of health and illness. He challenges Christians to express their concerns about these matters in ways that minister to the sick while giving expression to basic moral and religious convictions.

This is an important book for use within the congregation as well as among medical practitioners and ethicists. The ethical questions are developed in a way that will challenge much further discussion. The covenantal perspective is exciting and persuasive. Since contemporary issues of health and illness are ultimately moral and religious, studies such as Graydon Snyder has given us are critical if the church is to fulfill her mission.

Donald E. Miller, General Secretary
Church of the Brethren

Preface

My interest in health care ethics comes in part from personal involvement over several years in the administration of Bethany Hospital, located on the near West Side of Chicago, Illinois. The problems facing an inner city hospital raise sharply the issues of justice, distribution of resources, and the hopelessness advocating a traditional middle class ethic. At the same time, as a New Testament professor, I find that a faith stance becomes most clear when it takes form in a specific ethical context. I have often seen the covenant theology expressed in an ethic of peacemaking, but not so often in health care ethics. This study is primarily an attempt to explore the meaning of a particular faith stance in a complex ethical field.

I assume total responsibility for the ideas expressed here. From time to time there has been some collaboration with others, however. Some of the case studies and ideas came into focus because of a course on health care ethics taught with Donald E. Miller at Bethany Theological Seminary, in the Spring Term, 1986. That course ended with a consultation among students, faculty, and health care professionals. The ethics code of chapter 5 took shape in that consultation and was finalized at the Annual Conference of the Church of the Brethren in Norfolk, Virginia, 1986. A generous grant from the Brethren Health Foundation made possible the writing and publication of this book.

A number of people have helped me in different ways. I would like to express appreciation to Donald Miller, Bonnie Miller-McLemore, Nancy Poling, Linda Parrish, Jay Gibble, June Gibble, Tana Durnbaugh, James Kipp, Lee-Lani Wright, and Lois Horning Snyder. Special thanks are due Jeanne Donovan and David Eller of Brethren Press for their significant editorial assistance. Most of all I thank Nancy Wiles Holsey for her editorial assistance and her programming the manuscript for publication.

Graydon F. Snyder
Chicago Theological Seminary
November, 1987

1

Covenant Christianity

A doctor lets a severely impaired newborn child slowly starve rather than allow it to live for what would be a certain painful life and early death. Deeply religious parents refuse a blood transfusion for their dying child. A young boy with AIDS is not allowed to attend public school. A retarded young woman is made pregnant while institutionalized in a public facility. A ghetto child is kept off the kidney transplant list because her nonwelfare family lacks the $80,0000 needed for upfront payments. A husband is pardoned for putting his pain-racked wife to "sleep" with a fatal injection. Though the operation has never been successful, an intricate five organ transplant was performed on a child who otherwise had no chance of living. These and numerous similar situations exist across America. They are tough choices. What is right? What is wrong?

The problems of health care ethics in modern society are complex and manifold. A number of studies in this field are already available. It is not the intention of this study to bring new information. Rather, the purpose here is to examine some of the complex issues in health care from a particular Christian perspective, namely that of the believers' church. This tradition, generally regarded as the "left wing" of the Reformation, is sometimes termed the Free Church.

Unfortunately no single term suffices. Diverse modern denominations, including Brethren, Baptist, Disciples, and Mennonite bodies, to name a few, represent the believers' church. The reader will have to bear with references to a tradition that remains, at best, fuzzy.

Various attempts have been made to describe the theological and ethical concerns of this tradition, the most successful of which is Donald F. Durnbaugh's *Believers' Church* (1968). For the purposes of this exploration of health care ethics some important characteristics of the believers' church include:

1. Authority. At the center of faith for the believers' church lies the authority of the Bible, often primarily the New Testament. The meaning of the Bible and its guidance is determined by the faith community in study and prayer as they are led by the Holy Spirit. The faith community acts conservatively toward preserving its own tradition. But it also knows that the understanding of the text can grow and develop according to the social and political circumstances in which the church finds itself.

2. Voluntarism. Those church bodies using the term believers' church have invariably broken from a state church system or were originally formed as voluntary associations. Its members either are baptized as adults or understand that participation in the faith community entails an adult decision. This voluntary faith decision is known as discipleship. Disciples are those who decide to follow Jesus.

3. Mutuality. Because the faith community is guided by the authority of the Bible as understood by the community itself, the relationship between members becomes a central concern. Members treat each other with care, understanding, and respect. Historically, the believers' church has worked diligently at discipline within the fellowship. Sin is defined more as alienation than as evil deeds. Redemption is defined more as reconciliation than as liberation from demonic forces.

5. Peace. Since sin is seen as alienation, and God's redemptive action as primarily reconciliation, the faith community understands itself as an agent or ambassador of peacemaking. The problem of evil is not solved by destruction or even liberation, but by understanding and care.

Though this study attempts to express a health care ethic for one segment of Christendom, the believers' church, the theology expressed here may be characterized as *covenant theology*. While most groups within the believers' church tradition would adhere to covenant theology, that faith stance could hardly be limited to one segment of Christianity. The idea of covenant lies at the heart of biblical faith. The substance of God's covenant with us is stated in Genesis 12:1–3. That covenant was ratified with Abraham and his descendants in Genesis 15. The Hebrew scriptures describe how that covenant was expressed in Jewish history. Christians believe a new form of that covenant was created at the death and resurrection of Jesus. Historically the Bible has been named according to these two events: the Old Covenant and the New Covenant (Testament).

Because God's covenant is understood largely through the biblical witness many of the illustrations in this study will be taken from scripture. But other influences cannot go unnoticed. In 1648 a Protestant theologian, Johannes Cocceius, wrote a work on the theology of covenant. A follower of the Reformer John Calvin, Cocceius described a faith in God more dynamic and personal than the scholastic formulations developing in Lutheran Protestantism. Covenant or Federal theology not only influenced the Anabaptists from whom the Hutterites and Mennonites trace their origins, but more directly affected the believers' church through Protestant Pietism.

In modern times several major voices continue to understand the Christian faith in covenant terms. Josiah Royce, an American philosopher at the turn of the century, described Christianity in terms of universal community (*The Problem of Christianity*). More recently, sociologist Robert Bellah and others have decried the individualism which has come to pervade American society (*Habits of the Heart*). These influences continue to feed the conviction that a community or covenant ethic needs to be applied to the complex problems of our society.

When the term covenant theology is used in this study, it refers to a biblical theology which is also expressed in the anthropology of the biblical people. Relationships between God and the people are all important. That is also true of our relationships to each other. Truth is understood in faith terms rather than as facts or beliefs. It is more important to be faithful to God and each other than to be factually correct. In such a context of faith our lives are intertwined with others. In fact, we are formed by each other. We can and must be aware of who we are as individuals, but we also know that who we are has been formed by primary persons in our ongoing community. The writer of a book can only be an author if there are readers! A woman can be a mother only if there are children. A man can be a husband only if there is a wife. To put it directly, except for certain basic characteristics, such as gender, everything we are is a product of the formation process (1 Corinthians 4:7). Such an understanding of covenant is basic to this study.

A believers' church context and the idea of covenant have helped to form my understanding of health care ethics. Health is a factor of faith. Health is a factor of the human community. As such, this study assumes a psychosomatic understanding of health. It assumes that ill health can result as much from formation processes as from viruses or bacteria. It assumes that faith and trust are as important to good health as medicines and surgical procedures. It assumes that each of us and the faith community face tough choices as together we seek to understand and live out God's will.

Case Study

In the decade of the 1970s Bethany Hospital was a struggling hospital on the West Side of Chicago. About 40 percent of adults in the East Garfield Park neighborhood were unemployed. Welfare patients could run as high as 30 percent of occupancy at Bethany at any given time. It became clear the hospital could not remain as an independent institution. In 1981 the Evangelical Hospital System, a health care arm of the United Church of Christ, and the Church of the Brethren built a replacement hospital. Though a much superior facility, the new Bethany also has had difficulty serving a patient population that contained almost no third party insurance payments. The state allotment never covered the *per diem* cost of a hospital bed. Losses could run as high as $900,000 per month.

In the midst of these financial problems the state legislature decided to allot a certain number of "welfare days" to each hospital. For 1986 Bethany Hospital received a large allotment. Nevertheless in late November of 1986 the hospital had reached its limit. If patients on state aid were admitted in December there would be no state reimbursement. Financial advisors argued against admitting patients for whom there was no hope of reimbursement. If Bethany went bankrupt the hospital would be administered by the public sector or by a for-profit organization. Representatives from the United Church of Christ and the Church of the Brethren argued the hospital had an obligation to serve the poor regardless of reimbursement.

Questions for Discussion:

1. Would you expect a Christian hospital to develop policies different from public or for-profit hospitals? In what way?

2. How might a hospital or clinic sponsored by a believers' church make policy and health care decisions in a way that could be distinguished from other management groups?

3. Do you think Christians should be in the health care business? Why or why not?

2
Making Ethical Decisions

Making decisions about health care has become one of the most complex issues of our time. Most of us are aware of this fact—consciously or not—because every person faces, almost daily, some decision regarding health. In contrast to earlier years, even the simple process of eating a meal has become an ethical decision for many people. In recent years, proper care for the body through aerobics, exercises, jogging, or athletics has consumed the time and financial resources of countless Americans. At the same time, health care institutions, state governments, and particularly the federal government are spending millions of dollars to provide and develop even more health care resources and facilities. The decisions involved in the equitable use and distribution of these resources from a faith perspective constitute a major problem for persons concerned about health ethics. For many, such decisions are truly a matter of life and death.

This surge of health ethic concerns into the forefront of American personal and national problems is understandable. The most obvious reason has to do with resources or options. In the nineteenth century a person with heart problems did not have the choice between transplants, heart surgery, new valves, pacemakers or artificial parts. The resources simply were not available. Today there are many alternatives. How does one decide which option is best medically, which is fair for one individual in light of the needs of many, and how such alternatives can be financed? There is hardly any area of health care where dramatic new alternatives are not available. And the end is not in sight. Many believe that genetic engineering will change the nature of life as much as any research in recent times. And beyond genetic engineering are new horizons. The use of prenatal tissue to alter a diseased organ in adults, for example, will almost surely eliminate some diseases.

A second reason for the focus on health care ethics comes from the problem of a balanced distribution of resources and alternatives. Our society is conscious of the fact that new opportunities in health care ought not to be available simply for the wealthy or the powerful. This is particularly true, as in the case of kidney dialysis, when there are not enough resources to meet the need. Some persons cannot have dialysis and they will not survive. How does one make a decision? Who receives dialysis and who does not? On another level, organ transplants have become fairly commonplace, but there are not enough viable organs to save the lives of those who need hearts, livers, or kidneys. Who will receive the transplant? Some will live and some will die. How is that decision made? When there were no alternatives, the decisions were not difficult to make. But now that many alternatives are presented to us, the issue of justice becomes an extremely critical one.

A third reason for the growing concern for health care ethics lies in the nature of decision making itself, particularly with reference to the church and personal faith. Without overstating the case, it might be said that, a hundred years ago, health was an aspect of faith for that segment of the Christian world which held to a doctrine of original sin. Pain, illness, and death were understood as the tragic results of God's curse on Adam. Sickness and death were seen as

God's judgment on a sinful people. For those of us in the Free Church or believers' church tradition who have rejected, more or less, a doctrine of original sin, pain, illness, and death are understood more as the result of doubt and mistrust than as divine wrath. Put another way, illnesses are manifestations of psychological, sociological, and theological stress.

With the Enlightenment and the resulting demise of a universal understanding of faith, rational and scientific criteria emerged as the basis for all health care decision making. The advent of modern medicine at the turn of the century intensified this development with the result that modern health care is for the most part predicated upon rational and scientific terms. For example, in recent decades death has been defined as the cessation of the heart, the termination of brain waves, or the failure to breathe. People no longer think of life and death in terms of faith relationships. Consequently, in the absence of an understanding of basic life and death issues in the context of a covenant community, it has been necessary, for both legal and personal decision making, to make health decisions on solely scientific and rational bases. A major purpose of this book is to restore the element of faith to the center of health care decision making.

There are two ways in which people of faith make ethical decisions. Either a decision is made by some rational means or they adopt the ethical orientation of the Christian community of which they are a part. If my young child is about to purchase a toy weapon (which our church opposes) I might say, "We don't do that." If the child has reached the age of reflection, she or he may ask, "Why?" If the child does respond in that way then a rationale for the decision is necessary.

But a perceptive child might also ask, "Who are we?" In such a case the child is not asking for a reason, but for an identity. How are my values shaped by the community? Ethical decision making based on identity or group values is usually called "virtue ethics." We will call that "narrative" or "story ethic" and will deal with it in the third chapter.

Obviously, a person cannot always make decisions on the basis of his or her identity in the church. Some ethical problems may be quite complicated and require careful thought. In the remainder of this second chapter, we will deal briefly with some of the major considerations involved in health care decision making at a rational level. In the next chapter we will deal with narrative ethics and how such an ethical stance might affect decision making at a personal and community level.

There are two types of social theories which have greatly influenced ethical thinking in the western world. Contemporary reflection about health care ethics draws from these two ethical theories. A few words about them will be useful for later discussion.

The first of these is called *utilitarianism*. It was first proposed by an English philosopher and economist, John Stuart Mill (1806–1873). Utilitarianism is a way of making decisions on the basis of anticipated outcomes. To put it simply, we should act so as to bring the greatest benefit to the most people involved. Of course, the decision could be different from time to time. For example, should a young girl be told if she has a terminal case of leukemia? Normally physicians and family would share all information and the patient would be given access to all information regarding her or his condition. But it is possible that the girl would be happier in her last days if she were not consciously facing the threat of death. This could also enable the family to enjoy her presence for a longer period. A utilitarian might, therefore, argue for secrecy in this particular, special case.

There are two kinds of utilitarianism: *act-utilitarianism* and *rule-utilitarianism*. Act-utilitarianism occurs when a decision is made to do what you think is best for everyone involved. So, if the parents decide not to tell the girl dying of leukemia, their decision would be an instance of act-utilitarianism. But people object to the need for constant decision making. So over a period of time, it becomes accepted practice to say that certain ethical decisions will benefit most people most of the time. They might say something like: "generally speaking, everyone will be better off if we do this." When this line of rational argument is made, it is rule-utilitarianism. That is, a decision is made on the basis of the observation that most people are benefited when a certain type of decision is made. The rule-utilitarian would argue that everyone is generally better off if the complete truth about the patient's condition is known. In such a case the parents would then tell the little girl about her terminal leukemia.

As with any method of decision making, there are a number of serious problems with utilitarianism. In the first place, it is extremely difficult to take into consideration all of the persons who might be involved or affected by the decision. A family might decide what would be best for their own small group, but utilitarianism becomes very difficult at the state or national level. Secondly, outcomes of decisions are hard to predict. Something can always occur unexpectedly. A new factor or a new medical procedure can alter what appeared to be a sound moral decision.

Finally, many people do not sense the morality inherent in utilitarianism. Deciding according to context may appear as simple *pragmatism*. Pragmatism means doing what is practical and possible (based on observable consequences) in a given situation. A pragmatic decision may evidence no apparent moral structure or commitment.

Because of these weaknesses, many Christians prefer another type of decision making. The most viable alternative is what some ethicists call the *deontological*. The word comes from a Greek verb meaning "it is necessary." The morality of deontological decision making lies in a prior determination of what is right. Decisions will be based on clear absolutes. It does not necessarily ask about results. The German philosopher, Immanual Kant (1724–1804) was the major proponent of deontological thinking. Kant said that people should act in such a way that if their action were done by everyone, life would be perfect and satisfactory. Cases are not dealt with on their individual merit. Rather, the question is asked: "Should everyone act like this?" Suppose a wife has a husband who is dying of terminal cancer and is in great pain. How is she to think about whether to end his life and his pain? She cannot ask what would be best for everyone concerned (utilitarianism). Rather she needs to ask what every wife, or spouse, should do in similar circumstances (deontological ethics).

The deontological or "obligation" way of thinking is satisfactory to many Christians, because it offers moral direction which can be known in advance and thus can be taught. The Free Church tradition understands this way of thinking quite easily. For example, we could say that it is *always wrong* to take a life. That would mean that war is always wrong, and so is capital punishment, abortion, euthanasia, and mercy killing.

While there is a certain comfort in this way of deontological thinking, there are considerable difficulties as well. Since the deontological way of making decisions tends to place most of the moral responsibility on the individual, there may be some very strange, even inconsistent, results. For example, pro-life advocates make taking the life of a fetus a deontological prohibition. Yet for some strange reason they do not make the taking of life on the battlefield equally immoral. But from the standpoint of moral obligation, if the taking of life is wrong, then it is wrong across the board, before birth and after birth. It is clear that not everyone in the believers' church, for example, would agree with the prohibition against taking life under any circumstances. There are exceptions. Almost everyone would agree that sometimes it might be right to withdraw extraordinary medical means of life support.

The intense individualism which can be produced by an ethic of moral obligation arises because it is assumed that

each individual person knows what is right without considering how it affects others. Thus, the moral individual does not
necessarily need to engage in conversation with the community. This is clearly one of the problems facing the church
in our time. Those in the believers' church tradition are accustomed to making decisions as a faith community, at a local,
national, and international level, in light of the scriptures and
tradition of the Christian faith. As a faith community it is possible to take into consideration both the tradition as handed
down to the contemporary church, and the present, concrete
network of personal relationships.

Regardless of whether one is utilitarian or deontological,
there are four areas of health care ethics which need special
attention: autonomy, beneficence, nonmaleficence, and
justice. These are generally recognized by the law, the medical profession, hospitals, and health agencies as necessary
considerations. We will now turn to these four areas and indicate their importance.

Autonomy

As already suggested, the ethics suggested by Kant lead to a
type of individualism. One of the keystones of this ethic is
autonomy, a word which in Greek means literally "self rule."
The sense of autonomy is deeply rooted in American life—in
law, democratic traditions, and cultural self-understanding.
According to the Declaration of Independence and the Constitution of the United States, citizens have the inalienable
right to life, liberty, and pursuit of happiness. For many, the
laws of the land serve primarily to protect individual rights.

In health care ethics, autonomy primarily takes the form
of *informed consent*. This means that no one but the patient
has the right to agree to health care procedures. The
necessity for such a law and for such protection is immediately obvious. Many of us are old enough to remember
when cruel medical experiments were done on human

beings. The horror of such experimentation has led ethicists to conclude that no one has the right to perform a health procedure on a patient unless that patient has been informed of the procedure and its implications for his or her continued life. At the heart of the principle of autonomy is the belief in Western civilization that persons should be self ruled. But more than that, rules of autonomy prevent health care providers from practicing fraud or deception on an unsuspecting consumer. Furthermore, such laws force medical professionals to be self-regulatory in an effort to eliminate fraud. Even in the strictly regulated world of health care, however, desperate people can be highly gullible. The principle of autonomy makes it imperative that health care professionals state publicly all the information needed so that the patient can make the best informed voluntary decision.

This rule might at first seem reasonable. But even within this rule there are difficulties. The most obvious is the problem of competence. Is informed consent necessary for someone who does not have the individual competence to understand and act on the information? Or put another way, can procedures be initiated with a patient who is unable to give informed consent? People with a sense of moral obligation or a deontological perspective tend to say that consent is necessary, regardless. For example, if a person is being kept alive by extraordinary life support systems and cannot give informed consent, that support cannot be taken away. The principle of autonomy would insist that the person must give consent. But the patient cannot give it. The same would hold true for certain people in mental institutions.

The argument can also move in quite another direction. Let's assume that there is an age below which persons are unable to give informed consent. If a twelve-year-old daughter wished to give one of her kidneys to her mother in order to save the mother's life, most of us would not allow it. We would argue that the twelve-year-old daughter has no way of giving informed consent. The problem becomes stickier when dealing with infants. Normally health care personnel and parents must make all necessary efforts to save the life of an infant. But the decision to allow an infant to die is much more difficult. Informed consent cannot be given. The argument against abortion is most frequently a deontological argument. A fetus cannot give informed consent to its own death. Thus society says that where a person cannot be considered competent, medical procedures are extremely difficult to carry out.

Some of us believe that while the person who may be "incompetent" in terms of society's definition of individual competency, may in fact participate competently in the network of faith relationships. "Informed consent," then, would be a function of the community rather than a function based on individual competence. But in western, rational society, such a view is perceived as paternalism and as such is unacceptable. However the Free Church tradition may evaluate the principle of autonomy, we must reckon with the reality that American law as it now stands protects the individual as individual and thus reinforces the autonomy principle.

Beneficence

If the principle of autonomy is associated with deontological thinking, then the principle of beneficence is associated with utilitarian thinking. According to this principle, no procedure in health care should be initiated unless it promises to be of benefit to the patient. This is more than saying that no harm should occur (non-maleficence). The procedure must actually create some benefit for the person undergoing treatment.

For example, it has often been suggested that institutionalized retarded children might be used to test certain procedures. Such tests would be harmless. Yet it would be impossible to receive informed consent from the children (the problem of autonomy) and there would be no immediate benefit to them. For these reasons, most health care ethicists would say that we have no right to test procedures on retarded children even though benefit would be great to countless others.

Many Christians think of acting beneficially as a matter of love. But there is also a sense in which acting for the benefit of another is a moral duty. Ethicists think of it something like this:

1. Person *X* is at risk and has certain needs.
2. The action of another person, Person *Y*, is needed to alleviate the situation.
3. It is possible for Person *Y* to do this.
4. Person *Y* would not be at significant risk in performing the needed action.
5. The benefit to Person *X* would outweigh the risk to *Y*.

Ethicists say that under these conditions, Person *Y* has a duty to do an act of beneficence toward Person *X*. For example, if Person *X* is facing a life saving operation and needs blood of a rare type, then Person *Y*, who has that blood type, would have an obligation to give a blood transfusion. But if Person *X* is terminally ill and the intent of the transfusion is only to prolong life for a few hours, then Person *Y* could well say that the benefit to *X* is so small that it is not even worth the minor risk that he or she would take.

If an entire society or nation would follow this principle, there are moments when persons should act for the benefit of others. This is the basis for "good samaritan" laws, which are an attempt to protect those who would act beneficially. In health care ethics it might be whimsically said that health care professionals are obliged to act as minimally decent Samaritans.

Nonmaleficence

Whereas the principle of beneficence requires us to act for the good of another, or to prevent (or remove) harm, the principle of nonmaleficence requires us not to inflict evil or harm on another. At first this principle seems quite obvious, but such is not always the case. There is hardly any medical procedure which does not run the risk of inflicting some harm. Some of these are so obvious we hardly ever think about them. For example, to do a heart operation on a patient who does not have the strength to survive the operation would be a case of maleficence. The principle of nonmaleficence does not deal so much with the *intent to do harm* as it does with an *action which risks more harm than benefit.*

By law, a physician is required to take "due care." Just as it would be difficult legally to require someone to love another person, or act as a benefactor to another person, so it is difficult to legislate that health care professionals cure someone or make them better. There is always the possibility that a certain health care procedure will not work. But the law imposes strict standards regarding "due care." Minimally, the law says that health care people ought not to do harm. This, of course, serves as the basis for many law suits. It is in a sense the actualization of the old stories about the absent-minded surgeon who left a sponge inside the surgical opening. The physician who fails to better the condition of the patient may be considered an inadequate doctor. But the physician who does damage may be held accountable for what has occurred.

There are many instances when non-maleficence can hardly be avoided. Any medical procedure entails some risk to the patient. Most apparent are those cases where two lives are at stake. During times of delivery, the physician or midwife may have to decide for the well-being of the baby at the expense of the mother. Or, more often, the life of the fetus must be risked in order to ensure the safety of the mother. In such cases, the problem may not be solvable, and the physician or attending person must make a decision based upon prior values and professional judgments. Some religious groups, notably Roman Catholics, would call for the safety of the child, while others would call for the safety of the mother.

Justice

As we have already seen, the issue of justice has caused increased interest in health care ethics. The availability of medical choices has meant that the possibilities for treatment are more advanced, more widespread, and more complex. Who should benefit from these increased possibilities in health care techniques? The principle of justice concerns the appropriate distribution of health care resources. Many people suppose that health care resources should be distributed according to some commonly accepted pattern. We do agree, in American society, that some people justly deserve things that other people do not. For example, if someone has done the work for a high school diploma, then that person is given the diploma. We do not give diplomas to everyone simply because some have done the work. For most of us, that would not appear just.

But such a thesis applied too strictly can quickly become chauvinistic or racist. If we believe there is a hierarchy of justice, then it follows that resources should be distributed by some formula: according to individual need, or to individual effort, or to one's worth or contribution to society, or to merit. Each of these formulas have been tried by some major social system. A Marxist, for example, might wish to distribute resources according to need. A classical capitalist, on the other hand, might wish to distribute resources according to the person's contribution.

A system of hierarchy or class structure becomes so complex and unjust, many people have refused to use it. Many would say that in modern American society, medical resources are (or should be) equally distributed to everyone regardless of merit, contribution, or need. If there are not enough resources to go around, then the recipient would be chosen by chance. Thus under no circumstances would we say that this person will live and that person will die, *if* that choice is based upon a social distinction between the two persons. It should be done by chance.

Others strongly disagree and argue for some form of "socialized medicine" in order to allocate resources more evenly. Clearly the question of an equitable distribution of resources continues to be a major problem in health care for the years to come.

Case Study

A state legislature is considering a bill to establish community-based homes for retarded children and adults, who are now in four large institutions with a combined population of 7,600. The present set-up costs $55.8 million annually; the new one, which would provide one home for each fifteen residents would cost $70 million each year. The state representative who introduced the bill, with the backing of the state Department of Mental Health, the civil liberties union, and religious leaders, paints a dismal picture of overcrowding in the institutions and explains how the "cottages" would improve the quality of the inmates' lives. Opponents of the bill point out that the new plan would use up 2 percent of the state's budget while serving only 0.1 percent of its population. They argue that the proposed increase of $14 million could be used to buy hot lunches for all the state's school children and to provide job training to help people become productive members of society. The legislature should act, they believe, to promote the greatest good for the greatest number. At a public hearing, a physician points out that the money could be used to avoid mental retardation through prenatal diagnosis at a much lower cost than housing retarded children in institutions. (Taken from *Hard Choices*, p. 27)

Questions for Discussion:

1. Opponents of the bill for retarded children argue that such an expenditure would not promote the greatest good for the greatest number. Do you believe that should be an ethical principle?

2. Should the church promote the improvement of those who can contribute to society (through job training) more than care for those who cannot contribute much? Do you accept merit as a system of distributing our resources?

3. Do you agree with the physician that funds are better spent on prevention than in developing bandaids?

3

How Stories Shape
Decision Making

In the previous chapter two rational ways that people can make ethical decisions were discussed. One system calls for making decisions based on that which will serve the good of as many people as possible (utilitarianism). Another system calls for decision making on the basis of generally accepted norms (deontology). In both utilitarian and deontological ethical systems there are strong connections with the Christian faith. There is, however, another way of approaching ethics which relates more directly to the Judeo-Christian faith than these two. Many term the Judeo-Christian system a narrative ethic, while others call it virtue ethics. In current language usage, the word "virtue" often refers to an admirable quality rather than a basis for decision making; therefore, "narrative ethics" will be used in this book to refer to this system of decision making.

Despite what was stated in the first chapter, it is doubtful that people actually stop and reflect on an ethical decision. Many decisions must be made immediately such as a life or death action, or a decision during an operation. How are everyday decisions made quickly? People of faith make decisions on the basis of ethical values received from family and church. This formation of values occurs for a child on the basis of models and stories. Even the simplest stories convey moral or ethical values which provide the basis for action.

In what ways do these stories introduce a system of ethics? We will consider three ways by which a narrative enables ethical action: 1) the form of the story itself; 2) the actions and dialogues of the various characters in the story; and 3) the specific instructions given in the story.

The Form of the Story

First, the very shape of the story itself can teach what is important and what attitudes ought to be involved, without anything being said or described. For example, if my wife and daughter go with me to see a movie, they might observe the apparent male chauvinism in the film. When asked what suggests male chauvinism, they may not be able to respond. Their point is that women were ignored in the film. For a movie made in 1988 to ignore the issue of equality is in itself an ethical statement. Parents and educators who complain about many TV shows are right. It seems almost commonplace on TV that police narratives recognize the necessity of violence, if not killing, in order to curtail criminal activity. The ethics of reconciliation are often ignored. The very form of the police story makes an ethical statement even though nothing has been said deliberately. A hospital story which demonstrates unlimited possibilities for health care does considerable damage as well; since, in reality, possibilities are always limited. The form of the story seldom deals with the problem of equity in the matter of health care possibilities.

The Judeo-Christian formation of ethical decision making depends upon narrative. The revelation of God in the Hebrew scriptures is the narrative of the Torah, the first five books of the Bible. When we call Torah the law, we often assume that the core of the Torah consists of legal statements and requirements. But the Torah is primarily a story of faith, not a legal document. The moral guide for Jews, and subsequently Christians, comes in the form of a story. It will be demonstrated in later chapters that the Bible, particularly the Torah and the Gospels (the first four books of the New Testament) has become the basis for many of our health care decisions. That is certainly true of the synoptic Gospels (Matthew, Mark, and Luke). The Jesus of the Gospels consistently shows a concern not only for people who are excluded because of illness (such as lepers), but also shows a deep concern about their illness. Clearly the intent of Jesus is to cure the sick whenever possible (see Mark 1).

On the negative side, persons living in the twentieth century may be surprised at what appears to be a casual attitude by Jesus regarding certain ethical problems. For example, the story about Jesus cursing the fig tree hardly seems appropriate for a person concerned about a healthy world. But the Jesus of the Gospels was not an environmentalist. Similarly, the attitude of Jesus toward certain lifestyle issues that affect health seems somewhat surprising. The rather rigid dietary laws of John the Baptist appear more appropriate. Jesus, apparently, was accused of overindulging in wine and food. While this accusation was most likely not true, it does indicate that some lifestyle issues were not as important to the historical Jesus as they were to others of that time, or now.

The Characters in the Story

In addition to the way the story is told, ethical teachings are found in actions and dialogues of the story itself. This is very easy to see in the Gospels. Jesus healed a sick person almost any time one appeared in front of him. According to Mark 1, people crowded around him from morning to night in order to be healed. Jesus was a healer and the good health of persons was a concern of the creator God. This can be said with confidence about the man Jesus. But to be more faithful to the nature of narrative ethics, it should be said that those around Jesus understood him as a person concerned about health care, and they told the stories to emphasize that part of his ministry. Jesus not only acted to heal others, his words indicated his concern about health as well. Jesus of the Gospels, then, placed good health (wholeness) high on his list of human concerns. When faced with the needs of an individual as opposed to adherence to the law, he chose the health of the person (Mark 2).

If the ethical concerns of the storyteller and the community can be found in the hero of the story (Jesus, in the case of the Gospels), we can note that the opposite can often be found in the actions and the worlds of antagonists. Anti-heroes in a narrative are usually persons who exhibit undesirable characteristics; however, these characteristics may have nothing to do with the opponents themselves. For example, in recent American history Communists are frequently viewed as opponents. Their actions and words are interpreted as undesirable. It may not be true, but when a narrative or a TV show is developed, it is quite common to show Communists as uncaring, cause-oriented persons. Similarly, in the Gospels the antagonists of Jesus are frequently portrayed as persons who are in opposition to the concerns of Jesus and the narrator of the story.

Thus in the Gospel stories, the scribes and Pharisees often are more concerned about their understanding of laws, such as that of the Sabbath, than they are about the healing of persons. Or they may be more concerned about institutional control than wellness by insisting that people who are healed be examined by the priest and the temple officials. The Jesus of the Gospels does not deny the merit of laws and of institutions, but a comparison of Jesus' actions with that of the scribes and Pharisees indicates a high concern for the wholeness of the person on his part.

Jewish leaders ought not to be viewed as the only opponents in the Gospels. Frequently the disciples themselves are placed in opposition as well. The disciples were incensed by what seemed to them as the inappropriate action of the woman with the flow of blood when she came forward to touch Jesus (Mark 5:25–34). In another instance, they were unable to heal the boy with epileptic fits (Mark 9:14–29). Both of these accounts demonstrate a lack of concern and faith on the part of the disciples. It is interesting to note that it is often the marginal people who have the deepest concern and faith for the healing of persons. In fact, in Matthew 25 the common people are praised because they inherently know the right thing to do. That is to say, without reflection they acted out of the faith narrative of Israel and have helped people in prison and given cups of cold water to those who were in need. In contrast, other followers of Jesus cannot understand how they have missed doing what was right. One assumes they had determined what was the right thing to do and had acted correctly. The common people, on the other hand, acted out of narrative ethics without self-consciousness.

Specific Instructions in the Story

Because Judeo-Christians derive specific medical health care concerns from the biblical narrative, one can find summaries of that narrative that can be used as guides for health care ethics in general. For example, the Torah was summarized in the Ten Commandments. Admittedly, later generations have thought of the Ten Commandments as deontological or "obligation" pronouncements. But Judeo-Christianity has steadfastly refused to replace the wisdom of the Torah and the Gospels with specific laws, commands, and admonitions.

Let us look at a few of these indicators as they are found in the Ten Commandments, or Decalogue (Exodus 20:1–17; Deuteronomy 6:5–21). The biblical narrative ethic insists on loyalty to one God or, as translated into philosophical ethics, that we be guided by one purpose. So Christians living in the hope of the Kingdom of God act solely on that basis. That does not mean that concerns for research, financial solvency, institutional responsibility, and other loyalties cannot be recognized and given priority under the hope for the Kingdom, but the Christian finally makes a decision on the basis of that one loyalty to the living God.

The Judeo-Christian cannot reduce life to a thing or an it. Life consists of its living, and is made up of personal relationships. This is the heart of the covenant understanding of life. It is hard to overestimate the importance of this indicator. For example, the second commandment forbidding graven images means that life cannot be reduced to its mechanical, behavioral, or biological elements. Health care involves the wholeness of persons rather than simply the saving of a biological life. In terms of issues of birth, sex, and death, biological concerns need to be subordinated under personal concerns. Similarly, the person who needs health care can never be reduced to a thing or an object. Regardless of the illness or infirmity, each person stands in a covenant relationship with God and others. That relationship is the primary basis for any health care. Seriously damaged persons or handicapped persons may not be dismissed as irrelevant to society, or used as objects of research. Not only does everyone have rights, but everyone is a living person—and is to be treated as such.

Once this basic understanding has been assimilated, a number of other corollaries become self-evident. It is critical that all relationships be celebrated. Just as the celebration of the Sabbath defines our personal relationship to God, so with each other celebrations of key moments in the life of an individual or a family are absolutely necessary. Any major life-change requires a time for reflection. The most obvious changes are conception, pregnancy, birth, marriage, and death. But illness, leaving home for the hospital, long- and short-term debilitation, awareness of terminal illness, and loss of major friendships are also important moments. The biblical narrative ethic insists that we stop and celebrate these key moments in life as well. A health care system which does not allow times for reflection and concern has not really dealt with the patient as a person.

Along with the insistence that life is covenantal and that the progression of life must be celebrated comes the nearly absolute concern for the unity of the family and community. The formation narrative will mean nothing if the formation itself has been rejected. "Honoring your father and mother" means that persons have to come to grips with both their own origin and the narrative of their origin. Consequently, any health procedures must include one's family and com- munity. This obviously leads to problems with the principle of autonomy (self-rule).

A Christian ethic insists that family and close com- munity should be present. Health care procedures which vio- late the relationship of family do so at great risk. This is true not only of the family of origin, but of husband and wife, as the Decalogue points out (thou shalt not commit adultery). To be sure, the narrative of the New Testament indicates that disciples of Jesus may leave the family of origin. But that is done with the full awareness that a family is provided by the new community of faith.

All of this leads to an important indicator for any kind of ethic, but particularly for health care ethics. Because human personality is defined by its interaction with others, the prob- lem of death becomes far more important than either the issue of a person's right to life or the sanctity of human life itself. The individual's death is a death within the family and the community. Since the person who dies no longer interacts with the immediate family and community, the community and family themselves die in the process. To cause a person's death, or to let a person die, without recogni- tion of the fact that the community is diminished surely is the same as murder. Death cannot be avoided. Death is an event in a larger context. It is more than simply a heartbeat or the breath of an individual person. The reduction of a person to a thing who might live or die cannot actually be tolerated. In the Sermon on the Mount (Matthew 5-7) Jesus sharpens this issue when he says that the dismissal of a person as useless is equal to murder itself. The power of this indicator cannot be overestimated. This biblical understanding of death and dying in community has deeply influenced the nature of care of persons in western civilization, as well as forming the basis for hospital and, increasingly, hospice care.

The principle of autonomy suggests that the patient should know all the possible facts so that she or he can make a right decision. In the narrative ethic of the Bible, it is also indicated that information should be given and should not be falsified (Matthew 5:33-37). But in the case of the biblical narrative, the reason for speaking the truth differs significantly from the principle of autonomy. If the interrelationships of a healthy community are falsified, then correct decisions cannot be made. For example, the reason for "bearing true witness" in the family context is to allow the family to deal with the illness or a possible terminal situation. If that information is not shared, the community is living in a false situation and the family cannot possibly utilize the resources of the community for the illness. Jesus, in the Sermon on the Mount, insisted that this was true of all of life, not just certain key situations. For that reason, swearing an oath is improper, for to swear an oath indictes that there are other times when falsification would be appropriate.

As in the covenant kind of relationship we must never relate to another person as an it, so we must not relate to another in terms of their things or possessions. Consequently, we may not treat persons differently because they own more or fewer things. In the narrative of biblical ethics, justice depends upon the satisfaction of all persons involved in the community. It does not mean equity in distribution, but it does mean satisfaction. Goods cannot be used in order to receive greater benefit, nor should another person covet the possessions, prestige, or power of someone else in the community. In either case, theft or injustice will occur.

This indicator is just as powerful for our time. Not only does it deal with the issue of justice within the community, but it indicates that one ought not to use personal relationships for financial gain. For example, should a woman use her body's ability to conceive and give birth as a means of financial gain for herself and her family? Or can a man sell his ability to father a child?

Historical Narratives

Needless to say, the biblical narrative arose in different places at different times. Thus there are a variety of narratives within the Bible. There are, for example, four Gospels, each of which comes out of a particular time and place and contextual situation. It would be incorrect as well as inappropriate to claim that there is one clear ethical mandate in the biblical narrative. These differences have been cultivated by various religious traditions throughout the centuries. Even today, there are aspects of those differences in many denominations. For example, Evangelical Christians usually tell of powerful conversions with stories of people trapped in sin and released from that sin by the power of Jesus Christ on the cross. They speak of the miraculous nature of the conversion and the person's life because of the presence of Christ. Or, more charismatic individuals might tell stories of persons who were ineffective servants of God finding great joy in the gifts of the Spirit. As these stories are told they form persons who repeat patterns of "saving souls" or "receiving the Spirit." And, needless to say, one can find elements of these stories and others in the biblical narrative.

Traditionally, the believers' church narrative tends toward stories of service and hope. From my own background I know more stories of doctors who built hospitals in China, India, Africa, and South America than I do about evangelists who saved souls. Far more stories were told about persons who worked in disaster areas than about persons who "brought the Lord" to non-Christian areas of the world. This is not to say that evangelism is not a part of the Free Church tradition. But the Free Church story sees persons in a more wholistic sense. When the peace of God is brought to someone, it conveys a peace which includes health and justice.

Christians of many traditions in the twentieth century are frequently involved in health care activities. While no particular group has a monopoly on health care, the believers' church heritage does lead to intense care for persons in general and to the relationships within the faith community in particular. With this in mind, then, let us turn to an assessment of health care ethics in light of the biblical narrative.

Case Study

In the biblical world there was no known cure for lepers. When the disease was diagnosed, the victim was isolated from the rest of the community. Since disease was understood in a faith perspective the diagnosis was made by priests. In the unlikely event the leprosy was arrested, the victim was declared clean by the priests before returning to society. In Luke 17:11-19 there is the story of ten lepers who were watching Jesus from a distance (since they were unclean). Hoping to be cured, they called out to him for mercy. Jesus responded with a verbal affirmation and told them to present themselves to the priests. Once declared clean they could then return to their friends and families. Nine of the ten lepers did as Jesus directed, but one ignored the directive and the medical requirements. Knowing that he was cured, he rushed up to Jesus and the crowd. He fell at Jesus' feet and thanked him. Jesus praised him for his faith (in recognizing that he was well before he saw the medical authorities).

Questions for Discussion:

1. What may be learned from the narrative of the ten lepers?

2. What was Jesus' relationship to medical authority?

3. Why did Jesus praise the one who actually disobeyed him and ignored the proper procedure?

4

A Christian Approach to Health Care Ethics

The increasing complexity, cost, and potential options in health care will necessitate greater involvement in health care decision making by various social bodies. If the Christian community is to participate in that decision making, then it must think through its ethical stance in regard to this critical matter. Many denominations have worked through the questions of war and peace, economic injustice, and science and religion. But the church in general has been ill-prepared for the bombardment of health-related issues now facing it. The issues involved in such problems as the treatment of AIDS, surrogate motherhood, and genetic engineering are mind boggling from an ethical and spiritual perspective. It is imperative that Christian communities help their members understand basic guidelines which can be used in the wider community. For this purpose then, four major categories of ethics, autonomy, beneficence, nonmaleficence, and justice, will be reviewed from a believers' church perspective.

Autonomy

Though quite ancient as a virtue or principle, autonomy plays an important role in current medical ethics because of the events of our time. The specter of Nazi medical teams and personnel performing experimental operations on humans during World War II has mandated most of the world to insist that no one may be treated without her or his understanding or permission. There is no question about this concern. Most persons feel that it would be worth considerable sacrifice in other values in order to preserve the understanding that people are never to be treated as objects. At the same time there is a growing disenchantment with the paternalistic attitude of experts in American society, and health care people are no exception. Consumers of health care procedures feel that they have the right to know as much as the physician, explained in a language that they can understand.

As has already been indicated, there are clear problems with the concept of autonomy. From the point of view of biblical anthropology and most sociological thinking, the autonomous individual as frequently defined in the modern society simply does not exist. The human person, (*psyche* in Greek) comes into being through a complex process of corporate involvements. These involvements include, progressively, mother and father, siblings, extended family, peers, and then the wider community. It is a process of *formation.*

The human *psyche* is a marvelous intertwining of these various influences and encounters. A person who is capable of making rational, autonomous decisions is one who can find his or her identity in this complex process. Adults should have become sufficiently aware of their own personalities that they can reflect consciously about who they are. This awareness of self does not obliterate the formation process. It is well known that the biblical narrative maintains this unity of the person with the community. When one person does well the entire group is rewarded; when one person fails, the entire group is punished. The Israelite, Achan, who took forbidden items from the enemy, was punished not only by his own death, but by the destruction of all of his family and property (Joshua 7).

In the same way the men who tried to rape the angels in Sodom, and the men who raped the mistress of the traveler in the area of Benjamin, brought down the wrath of God and the tribes on all of them. The assumption is that such irregular behavior could not have occurred unless the community itself had become defective in the process of formation. Since the individual *psyche* is created by the community, a defect in the community and its formation must result in the defect of the individual. This is the meaning of God's curse on Adam. It is not to say that through one individual, lust or sin entered into the world. Rather, it is that through Adam a defect in the community occurred which cannot be erased except in Jesus Christ. Indeed, the good news of Jesus Christ is that the fault of formation can be overcome by the action of God among the people of God.

Once it is understood that humanity is not composed simply of persons who cooperate with each other or who are intertwined through various networks and systems, but actually results from the creation of the individual *psyche* out of the total, then the issue of autonomy takes on a different character. Autonomy in the rationalistic, individualistic sense of the word does not exist. The Judeo-Christian ethic understands that the individual makes decisions on the basis of formation in any case. So it would be better for the community central to the person's formation to be present with that person when health care is needed, both in terms of care itself and in terms of a sharper decision-making process.

Solid health decisions ought to be made by the individual in the presence of the individual's immediate family, his or her faith community, and a key peer person—in light of the scripture and in light of the best medical knowledge possible. For this reason, many health care experts now suggest that the person needing health care assistance be offered a support community that consists of the doctor or skilled health care worker, a pastor or spiritual leader, family members, and representatives from the local church. In this way, the patient can receive the benefit of medical advice, the power of a particular faith tradition, and the best thinking of the family in a wholistic decision-making setting.

Non-Maleficence

The Judeo-Christian narrative or story begins with the process of ordering. This may take the form of a creation story itself, such as in Genesis 1–3, or it may take the form of an explanation for why certain events are occurring, such as the conflict with Pharaoh in the early chapters of Exodus. The ordering process or God's creating is expressed both in narratives of the creation of the world and in stories which tell of God's saving acts. As the biblical story develops it then shifts to the end time. It expresses in various ways what is expected to happen, what is hoped will happen, or even what is happening. This may be expressed in formal "apocalyptic" or end-time passages, such as in Mark 13, Revelation 20, or Isaiah 55.

Throughout the biblical narrative there are numerous expressions of peace and reconciliation and the possibility for a new relationship between humanity and creation itself. Most of the story, however, deals with the time between creation and the end time. It is in this tension between the beginning and the end where decisions have to be made in light of where God's people have come from and where we are going. In terms of biblical theology the narrative is a promise and fulfillment. The beginning point of the story is the promise of God and the end point is the fulfillment of that promise. The narrative about in-between times is a description of how people live between the creation and the end.

An examination of most of the narratives of the Bible shows that they move between these two poles. For example, a major story in the Hebrew Scripture, the ascension of David to the throne, begins with God's promises to David that he will become the king. The story then builds by telling how the author believes the promise was fulfilled. The next story describes the succession to David. God promises that there will always be a son of David on the throne and so the story progresses in such a way as to show the reader how the succession occurred in Solomon. The behavior of the principal actors in this narrative might shock us in terms of more absolute ethics, but the material is designed to show that even unethical behavior, while not exemplary, can become a part of the fulfillment of the promise. Frequently, as in the story of the relationship of David, Bathsheba, and Uriah, the narrative may depend on an immoral action, but the fulfillment is achieved only because of the grace of God.

So it would be quite unfair to say that the action of the people of the Bible serves as an example of how one moves between creation and end time. The major message of the Bible is that God has granted us the taste of the nature of the end time even though we act in such a way as to oppose the coming of the end. In other words, the intention of God pulls us toward that end whether we act appropriately or not. The time between the beginning and end, creation and end time, is one in which the pull of the end time creates a possibility which the actor in the drama does not intend. Because of God's will for the end, God may act gracefully toward the ill-conceived actions of persons who are involved in the narrative.

Life in the "between times" may be characterized as conservative toward creation and radical toward the end time. The Christian thus has a dual responsibility: to act in such a way as to preserve the creation and to act in such a way that the radical nature of the Kingdom of God may be possible now. What some today would call "non-maleficence" actually corresponds to the Christian understanding of creation. The health caregiver is not to take action that would harm the client. But the Christian understanding is much broader. The Christian ought not to harm what God has created. This is not so much to instill a sense of awe or obedience. Rather, the emphasis of the doctrine of creation lies in the affirmation that all of God's creation is good.

There are basically two elements that compose the Christian's attitude toward creation. The first of these is the need for security in the formation of personhood. Second is a positive concern for the created universe. Let's elaborate.

In the believers' church it is assumed that the human personality develops in the context of the natural family, the closest community, and then, eventually, the faith community. As already noted, the assumption is that health derives largely from the integrity of these relationships. When personhood is threatened or alienated, then ill health can easily follow. While the Christian is interested in service and deeply concerned about people who have come into ill health, the Christian also recognizes that ill health was not intended in the creation. Continuing the goodness of creation, then, becomes as important as healing the broken. For example, an alarming number of children today are found to be abused in their primary family situations. While it is important to help these children, even to the point of finding them foster homes, the Christian ethic understands that the real solution to this problem lies in the development of better family life—the primary location for "person" formation.

In another case, that of abortion, there has been much debate between those who support the right to life and those who support the right of choice. However difficult this may be, the Christian must recognize that the death of a fetus is not the primary issue. A society in which women can be abused, or in which men and women can conceive children they do not want, ought not to exist. The Christian is as concerned about the loving relationship between men and women as the life or death of an unborn fetus.

Since health depends upon formation, then people of faith will invariably act conservatively on the formation process. The Christian who is concerned about health issues looks with deep concern into such problems as surrogate motherhood, sperm banks, *in vitro* conception, abortion, incest, child abuse, care of those imprisoned, care of the handicapped, and care of the elderly. From a Christian perspective, all of these concerns may point to an underlying disease in our personal formation.

Just as the believer acts conservatively toward formation of the person, so also does he or she acts conservatively in relationship to the creation. Christians "refrain from doing harm" to their own personhood (including their bodies), to the environment, and to the whole of creation itself.

It is difficult to argue for a personal Christian ethic. All ethics depend upon relationships to one another and to the created world. Still, there are actions often referred to as personal that have actually become concerns for society at large. Consider, for example, the abuse of drugs. This affects not only one's personal body but also life within the community, relationships with family and community, and the economics of the locations where drugs are manufactured, distributed or sold, and used. Drug abuse may result in dependency and debilitation, cancer, AIDS, and other serious medical problems. While Christian groups may feel the need to build sanitariums for victims of substance abuse, the Judeo-Christian attitude toward creation would obligate believers to work toward preventing the causes. A New Testament parallel might be leprosy. Jesus did not build caves and camps for the lepers, but offered them a cure, that of wholeness.

On a more public level, the misuse of nuclear fission, insecticides, brown coal, lead, and gasoline, are all issues which affect the natural environment in which we live. It seems clear that we have created the conditions that give rise to many of the diseases we need to cure.

A recent study indicates that had we used as much effort and finances for the prevention of cancer as for the cure of cancer, we might have saved thousands of lives. This approach represents the Judeo-Christian conservative attitude toward creation.

Beneficence

In narrative ethics the end of the story, which indicates the final desired outcome, does not occur necessarily on the last page. Somewhere in the story the faith community will point to what it expects. In the case of the Bible, the last book, the Revelation of John, tells of a New Jerusalem coming down from heaven. Isaiah 55 and 65 also describe what the end time will be like. Those who look at the Christian story from a strictly rational perspective often speak of such expectations of the end as misguided or false hopes. They regard the prophets and Jesus as persons, trapped in a Jewish time-frame, who expected an end to history that never came. Sometimes such persons view the ethics of the biblical narrative as "interim ethics." These are of little value however, since we all "know" the world is not coming to an end. Similarly, those people who believe they can discern an actual calendar or a day when the end will occur have misread the biblical material.

The story of the Bible raises in us an anticipation of the end time as described in Revelation 21 or Isaiah 65. The Christian has a permanent end-time expectation or hope. Armed with that kind of confidence, the believer acts radically toward the future. The love ethic which calls for beneficence leads the faith community to much more than what some have humorously called "the minimally decent Samaritan." The Christian does not work for the *benefit* of other persons but, rather, the *wholeness* of the other persons. *Agape* love, God's love, does not count the cost to the giver. It is a radical stance toward the end time. Faith in the nature of the end time not only calls for radical action, but such a faith makes radical action possible. The Jesus of the Gospels called on us to sell all we have and give to the poor, to turn the other cheek when attacked, to love the neighbor as ourselves. These radical demands are possible only in light of the intense expectation of an end time. And by end time Jesus meant the "breaking in" or the presence of the Kingdom of God among God's people.

The issue of radical hope becomes a critical issue for health care professionals. For example, in terms of so-called "lifeboat" ethics, the Christian probably is unable to make a negative decision. In the lifeboat analogy there are ten people with food enough for only nine. The question is, who among the ten should be thrown overboard? In terms of radical hope, the Christian cannot sacrifice one life for the sake of the nine others. The wholeness of all ten are equally important. This question becomes very difficult when applied to a hospital operating in a primarily indigent area. If the hospital will be paid for only a certain number of indigent or welfare patients, should the hospital ever turn anyone down because no public payment will be available for that person? Or is the Christian hospital obligated to treat anyone who comes to the door? The radical hope of the Christian would suggest that everyone should be treated, even if this raises the issue of the financial future of that hospital. On the other hand, is it appropriate, or even Christian, for a hospital to "commit financial suicide"? Will that not make the situation of the community worse than it was before? The destruction of caring institutions leaves wholeness in the hands of the "for-profit" sector.

Health care professionals face the same issue when they must decide whether to treat persons with a disease that is contagious. A key issue of our time is and will continue to be the treatment of persons with AIDS. To what extent should health care professionals risk contracting the disease themselves? Will public knowledge of such treatment make other patients shun them? What is the responsibility of a hospital? Will treatment of AIDS patients create a risk for other patients? Will the general public shun a hospital that treats persons with AIDS? From a Christian narrative perspective, faith heroes have indeed taken such risks. In the New Testament, Jesus healed the lepers. He apparently did not avoid touching them. Throughout history, Christians have led the way, at no small risk, in the establishment for the care of lepers or tubercular patients. Christians will do the same with persons who have AIDS. The issue is even more complicated because persons who have AIDS may have contracted the condition in a way alien to the generally accepted Christian lifestyle. Christians, with their radical hope, can never say no to a person in need. Love leads to much more than beneficence.

Justice

The Judeo-Christian sense of justice does not quite match that of the secular ethicist. While Christians would not find it right to give preferential treatment or to make decisions on the basis of merit, neither do they find strict equality an appropriate principle. In the biblical story justice refers to the peace (*shalom*) of the faith community. That means that the individual is received in the faith community as a legitimate and full member. The ultimate expectation is that each person finds her or his role satisfactory. It is never understood that people have the same role in the faith community or that people are equally endowed to play every role. Every analogy of community life in the Bible expresses this view. In Paul's analogy of parts of the body (1 Corinthians 12), he explicitly indicates that each member is to be understood as a critical part of the body, but each plays a different role. Furthermore, each member is treated differently. The early church stressed the *quality of satisfactory participation* in the faith community rather than *equal treatment* of each individual or equal distribution of resources and honors. This may seem odd to many modern readers who wish that early Christians like Paul would have been more interested in the abolition of slavery in the Roman Empire than in the acceptance of all persons in the faith community (see the letter to Philemon).

The reason justice is so defined becomes obvious in light of the Judeo-Christian understanding of humanity. Equal involvement in community is a primary concern for Judeo-Christianity because that is where formation of the person occurs. A person cut off from the community dies. When, for social or health reasons, people are isolated, then death has occurred. The concern for a person's health does not reside primarily in equality but in the dynamic involvement of everyone in the corporate life.

Since formation differs from person to person and since people are at different levels of their life span, it is reasonable to suppose that people are not interested in identical treatment. For example, a person with a kidney ailment might prefer not to take any radical measures, or rather, might prefer a transplant, or some form of dialysis. Such decisions would be made on the basis of age or placement in life. It would be wrong to assume that every person considers a lengthy continued life, at any cost, to be the optimum choice. Of course the problem of kidney dialysis places the issue of justice squarely in front of us. The Federal government spends $20,000 a year on each of 6,000 patients. Should the entire $120,000,000 be spent in other ways? Many countries cannot afford the kind of expenditures that the United States makes on dialysis. In Cuba, for example, a person with terminal kidney dysfunction is given a transplant when possible. Dialysis itself is not available.

There are segments of the population which do not receive equal treatment. To what extent should Christians insist on total health coverage for the indigent or the elderly? Are there then persons in society who should be responsible for his or her own situations? Should those persons who take risks in their own lifestyle also be granted assistance by the total community?

In my view the faith community must not allow injustice. Marginalized elements of society such as the unemployed, the indigent, and the elderly should receive adequate health care. That means subsidizing health care for some people, seeking a higher percentage of compulsory health insurance for all people, or even advocating some form of a national health care program. At the same time, the faith community would not wish to force programs on those who chose by their lifestyle or convictions to care for their health in other ways. The faith community opts for equal opportunity, but not compulsion.

Case Study

Janet P., a practicing Jehovah's Witness, had refused to sign a consent for blood infusions before the delivery of her daughter. Physicians determined that the newborn infant needed transfusions to prevent retardation and possible death. When the parents refused permission for these transfusions, a hearing was conducted at the Columbia Hospital for Women to decide whether the newborn infant should be given transfusions over the parents' objections. Superior Court Judge Tim Murphy ordered a guardian appointed to sign the necessary releases, and the baby was given the transfusions. During the hearing, Janet P. began hemorrhaging, and attending physicians said she needed an emergency hysterectomy to stem the bleeding. Her husband, also a Jehovah's Witness, approved the hysterectomy but not infusions of blood. This time Judge Murphy declined to order transfusions for the mother, basing his decision on an earlier DC Court of Appeals ruling. Janet P. bled to death a few hours later. Her baby survived. (This case is based on a news report by Martha M. Hamilton in *The Washington Post*, November 14, 1974. It was prepared by James J. McCartney.)

Questions for Discussion:

1. At what point should the value of an individual life (Janet P.) outweigh the convictions of her religious community (Jehovah's Witness)?

2. Should the court have made a judgment about Janet P. on the basis of criteria other than informed consent? Should she have been allowed to die because she would not give consent? What other criteria could have been used?

3. Do you consider the issue of a transfusion a covenant matter? Was Janet P. forced to withhold consent because she valued relationships with her faith community more than she valued her life?

4. What health care decisions would you hesitate to share with your faith community?

5. On what basis could the judge decide transfusions could be given to the baby, but not to the mother?

5

A Health Decisions Code

The relationship between the biblical story and a code for health care decisions is one of the most confusing of all issues. A code or creed states in a public form what the narrative has said to people who believe in and operate out of a given story. It is appropriate for people to create codes and creeds out of narrative statements because it is almost the only way in which a larger public can understand why a group of people act or believe as they do. Codes and creeds can often help some people grasp more easily the general intent of the story. The problem comes when people believe that the creed or the code itself is the faith of the community. That is not and dare not be true. A moral code does not have the ability or power to transmit the concerns of the community at large. The power of a creed to form ethical behavior is minimal compared to the power of the narrative.

The narrative creates the person, with or without compliance to creeds or codes. Within Christian history people have created creeds and codes as a means of forcing unity within the corporate community, and as such they have been the cause of harassment, even to the extent of torture and martyrdom. People in the Free Church tradition are uneasy about codes and creeds for this reason. Direction for life comes out of the primary story, which is why, in the Sermon on the Mount, Jesus says, "You have heard that it was said of old, but I say unto you." That is, people had made a code of the faith story in the Hebrew scriptures. Jesus did not disagree with the faith narrative, the *Torah* or law. To the contrary, he felt that the entire narrative would be fulfilled. Jesus did disagree with the use of codes and creeds to enforce a faith or a morality which was more appropriately transmitted through narrative. Had that been true people still would have acted "from the heart" and not out of "fear of the law."

Yet, from time to time, faith communities have also found it useful to express in pronouncements and resolutions what they believe. For example, the National Council of Churches has issued significant statements on genetic engineering. Only recently the Roman Catholic Church issued important statements regarding surrogate motherhood and artificial insemination. My own Brethren tradition has adopted statements on aging, AIDS, genetic engineering, abortion, and similar issues. Other believers' churches have expressed themselves as well. When, as is frequently the case today, new medical possibilities and questions arise, it is necessary for the church to speak to those issues. Allow me to state again, however, that the ethic is found in a relational formation of personhood through stories, not in a pronouncement or in moral codes.

With that caution in mind, we turn to the possibility of a health decision-making code for the Free Church. The following sample statement was formulated by members of several believers' church bodies. The final form (with only minor editorial revisions) came out of a meeting of health care professionals, patients, church people, theological students, and seminary professors in the spring of 1986. It is given here, with my commentary, in the hope that it will guide church leaders and congregations in the formation of support groups for persons making health care decisions.

1. The person receiving health care assistance and procedures should be fully informed about the intended care, and should participate in all decisions made.

Even though the covenant style church is community-oriented, whenever possible health care assistance should be given to an individual only with the permission or knowledge of that individual. The sense of community does not engulf the individual, but recognizes that an individual acts in a corporate context. The faith community might differ from current public practice when the patient is not actually competent. Because of the sense of autonomy, the public realm is immobilized when the recipient of the health care is incapable of hearing the information, understanding it, or making a decision. In such a case the believers' church tradition would recognize that an appropriate group of persons could act on behalf of the incompetent person. So, for example, a hospital ethics committee composed of physicians, nurses, and faith community could help the family make the decision to cease the extraordinary measures used to preserve a comatose person (see chapter twelve).

2. Concern for autonomy ought not to outweigh ordinary procedures for decision making in conversation with the faith community.

The covenant-type faith community recognizes that a person has come to a specific point in life in relationship to significant others. This part of the code protects that involvement. It is not so much to say that a committee or group could act on behalf of the incompetent person, but asks that health care people recognize the necessity of a group decision. The people who have helped form an individual and continue to live close to that person would reasonably be involved in the decision-making process. One thinks particularly of the faith community (the congregational health care committee), the family, and the pastor. Such persons need not be consulted regarding health care procedures, but they should at least be provided a normal role in the decision-making process. Should a middle-aged person opt for a transplant? Should an older person agree to a life-threatening operation? Should a couple hire a surrogate mother? Should a fetus be altered? All of these are faith questions which involve not only the person but the person's social environment. For this reason persons should be identified within the faith community who are capable of either giving wise advice or at least sharing with those who face difficult health care decisions.

3. The faith community should develop means for members to participate as informed persons in health care decision making. The responsibility of the church is to suggest and make available various options.

Given the complexity of health care decision making, various people not only should serve as a support group for its members, but at least some members of the congregation should have more than a passing knowledge about the current status of medicine, health care, and preventive procedures. Decisions should be made within the faith community in light of the Christian tradition and the best information from the human sciences. A small congregation may opt simply for a group of people who make it their vocation to be aware of health care issues. Such a group would not only support members in their decision-making process, but would be advocates of preventive measures and health care lifestyles. A larger church might have, in addition to a particular program such as the congregational health care committee, specific health interest groups, or even a church nurse program.

4. The faith community should provide support for the decision of the individual, made in the context of conversation with the community, regarding the initiation, continuation, or cessation of treatment.

This code makes more explicit what has been said through the first three statements. The Christian is to make statements on treatment on the basis of the best knowledge possible from health care experts as well as from the point of view of life as understood by the faith community.

5. Responsible ethical decisions should be made on the basis of information provided by health care experts and on the basis of the understanding of life offered by the faith community.

It should be understood that health may depend on faith and trust as expressed by one's support group, but that in no way replaces the technical knowledge of health care professionals. Christians believe expert medical skill should be used in a faith context.

6. The faith community should be an advocate for its members regarding the preservation of God's creation, particularly in matters of ecology.

The faith community should be more than a support system or a decision-making system. It should also take an advocacy role. We have already indicated in chapter four that the Christian community will become activists in regard to environmentalism, lifestyle issues, preventive medicine, proper exercise, proper food consumption, and health education. While there may be right and wrong approaches to these matters, the church ought not to be awkward or embarrassed about advocacy. At this point the larger faith community ought to assist the local congregation in the style and nature of its advocacy.

7. The faith community should be an advocate for its members regarding a lifestyle which prevents health disorders.

As indicated in the sixth code, the faith community should act clearly in regard to personal lifestyle. Many of the believers' church communities have already taken stands on the use of drugs or foods that could do physical or mental damage. All local congregations should make this a point of Christian education, not only for the individual but as a social policy expressed in community legislatures.

8. The faith community should help its members understand increasing technologies in health care, but balance them against the faith meaning of life. That is, life and death should be understood as matters of faith, not simply matters of physical life and death.

The faith community does not operate out of any rigid sense of revelation. Any person making a health decision should take into consideration the technical issues (understood as part of creation) as well as the faith issues. In an increasingly complex technological world, the faith community should understand one of its tasks as the education of its members about technology. We need to live by a faith perspective that is informed by technological advances. An understanding of God's revelation goes alongside an understanding of God's creation. The faith perspective needs to be restored. Issues of life and death, health and illness, should come to be understood primarily in the faith context.

9. The gospel story of the death and resurrection of Jesus Christ leads the faith community and health care professionals to sacrificial giving of ourselves, health services, and health resources for the common good of suffering humanity.

The main elements of the gospel story do not assume the paradise of Eden, nor the peace of the end time. We live in a world which is complex and broken. Unfortunately we cannot idealize issues of life and death, or health and illness, in terms of the Garden of Eden or the New Jerusalem. The gospel story speaks of God's self-giving in Jesus Christ and the unlimited possibilities that come from that understanding of life. The problem of health in the faith community is not just a rational process; there is also considerable hope because of the death and resurrection of Jesus Christ. We can and will be surprised by the grace of God and the power of faith. Therefore we, as a faith community, not only expect and pray for the grace of God, but we also act graciously. We, like Jesus, give ourselves to the world in the hope that health will prevail.

10. Quality of life is to be valued along with protection from injury so that health care resources for education and prevention are to be balanced with crisis medical care.

This code stresses particularly the need for prevention and education. Christians are called upon to respond to crises and disasters. But we ought not to consider this our primary obligation. Believers ought to be sufficiently aware of trends that they can act in such a way as to prevent ill health.

11. Health care resources should be available to all person including the poor, minorities, the elderly, and the oppressed.

The issue of just distribution has been discussed in the previous chapter. While governmental agencies and health institutions may be aware of justice issues, it is important for the Christian community to continue advocacy for those who are overlooked or abandoned. Such a concern is deeply rooted in the Christian tradition. The early church was noted for its concern about persons on the periphery. The same concern for the widows and orphans can be seen in the Hebrew scriptures.

12. A system of health is needed that is not governed primarily by profit, but primarily by the fair distribution of health care to the whole community.

It may be that "for-profit" medical institutions are incapable of acting out of ethical norms suggested here. It is important for the faith community to continue to support private, church, or synagogue oriented health care institutions. If the concerns of the faith community are to be expressed, there will need to be health care institutions that express them.

13. A minimum level of health care is a right of all people.

The western world has adopted a privatistic understanding of personal rights. The Constitution of the United States protects the rights of all citizens. During this century the countries of western Europe and the United States have developed other types of personal rights for their peoples. Among these, the right to health and health care, however, has not been stated as such. The faith community believes that every person has rights to preventive medicine and health. As we have indicated already, this does not necessarily mean equity in distribution. Individuals could have different requirements at different stages of their life and at different places.

The faith community could argue though that certain elements or "rights" are non-negotiable. In health prevention, for example, it can be said that every person has a right to an environment that is free of harmful air and water pollutants and of radiation. In terms of health, would we not agree that everyone has a right to prenatal care and birth care? Yet the issues quickly become complicated. The extent to which everyone has the right to extraordinary means of preserving life, through very expensive aids, remains to be decided. If the patient is uninsured and/or financially destitute some may question their right to treatment in life-threatening emergencies. But clearly everyone has a right to expect certain minimal standards of health care.

14. Arbitration and mediation are to be encouraged as alternatives to law suits that are increasingly costly to everyone.

On the practical side, a major reason for the inaccessibility of minimal health care has been caused by the rising costs of insurance and legal fees. In order to establish better health care for everyone, the church needs to encourage arbitration in such cases rather than court battles. The faith community should work in each state for the kind of legislation that would limit legal suits, while still protecting the public from poor medical practices. At the same time, the faith community believes that true biblical justice can take place only through reconciliation. While the state might reasonably dispense justice, normally it cannot bring about reconciliation. The believers' church tradition is that such reconciliation ought to occur not only within the faith community, but also within society as a whole. For this reason, the church should advocate the use of reconcilers and arbitrators who seek to avoid costly, destructive legal suits.

15. The various levels of health care providers are encouraged to work as a team rather than as competitors.

Not only should the faith community call for wholistic health care, that is, care for the person as created as well as the person that is intended; it should also call for society as a whole to utilize its resources in a team effort. Resources, such as the number of clinic and hospital beds available, should serve all the health needs of the community—including drug abuse and AIDS patients.

16. The health and spiritual needs of health care providers should be recognized and cared for.

Many in the church have a tendency to suppose professionals are self-perpetuating and super-human. That is not true. Persons dealing with health, severe illness, and terminal illness are under incredible stress and the faith community needs to support them with extraordinary measures. Support groups need to be created for persons in health professions.

Case Study

James N. and his spouse Sarah lived in Harrisburg, Pennsylvania. James had already retired with a modest pension while his wife Sarah still worked in a social service agency. Sarah developed breast cancer. A radical mastectomy arrested the cancer and she was in remission for three years. Then the cancer reappeared in her chest and in the lymph nodes. She was forced to quit her job. The couple was left with only James' moderate, fixed income. After chemotherapy Sarah's physician agreed that her prognosis was not good. He suggested a bone marrow transplant. The procedure would be experimental and would cost about $100,000. Yet it was her only chance to live. Sarah and James were undecided. Because of the umbrella style insurance, a bone marrow transplant would take all their savings and seriously deplete the pension. Sarah and James were strong members of the Pilgrim Church in Harrisburg. They took their dilemma to the faith community.

Questions for Discussion:

1. At what point does the cost of health care begin to outweigh the value of "more time"?

2. Do you think James and Sarah were right in approaching their faith community about their decision? Discuss your reasons for your answer.

3. Given the code in this chapter what do you think the Pilgrim church group should say to James and Sarah?

6

The Meaning of Life

Life is defined for the faith community as life in covenant relationship, and persons are understood in terms of the formation that created them. In the Judeo-Christian world formation, family life and education are absolutely primary concerns. One gives significance and meaning to others and receives significance and meaning from others. We have seen how the Ten Commandments stress the meaning of this relationship. With some exceptions, the entire Bible protects this formation process. In 1 Corinthians 7:4 Paul says that the wife is in authority over the identity of the husband and the husband is in authority over the identity of the wife; therefore, they owe each other mutual relationship. Those relationships can cross over even cultural and religious boundaries (1 Cor. 7:12–17). Within the context of such a family, children are formed as faithful children (1 Cor. 7:17).

Seen from a covenant perspective, life begins when the formation of a new person begins. The same is true of the end of life, which comes when formation can no longer occur. While the faith community recognizes this, the medical community and the public generally do not. It becomes necessary for the faith community to be in dialogue with the technical or public community in order to preserve and foster the covenant understanding of life.

Many of the major issues in medical ethics center on the problems of birth and death. In light of previous discussion, some of the issues regarding birth will now be considered.

Conception

The Judeo-Christian God is in no sense a static entity. God is the source of creation and Jesus Christ is the agent of creation (1 Corinthians 8:6). When the New Testament speaks of Jesus Christ as with God from the beginning (John 1:1–14; Colossians 1), it is saying that the God revealed in the Bible was from the beginning a God who was and is creating the other. The very nature of mutuality is to be creative. While there may not be a one-to-one equation between creation and procreation, it is extremely difficult to read the entire Bible without drawing such a conclusion. Certainly the issue of childlessness is a significant theme in the Bible. It has been said that in the biblical narrative women without children have not been fulfilled. A more helpful approach would be to say that a mutual marriage has not been consummated until it has become creative. For this reason women such as Sarah, Rachel, Hannah, and Ruth seek assistance from the Lord in the development of a family. In any case, the process of conception, giving birth, and formation are highly valued and protected in the Judeo-Christian scriptures.

Consequently, a purely biological understanding of conception does not satisfy most Jews or Christians. The conception of a child is an act of mutual covenantal agreement. It may be going too far to say that the conception of a child must always be an act of love. Yet it is on this basis that some people would rule out surrogate motherhood or artificial insemination.

The Judeo-Christian view of sex does not allow sex to be reduced to a mere biological relationship. Because the relationship between husband and wife is covenantal, intimacy can express that covenant without requiring the possibility of a child. For this reason Protestantism in general, and the Free Church in particular, does not oppose contraception. However, sterilization raises a different problem. From the believers' church perspective, sterilization after a family has been developed enables the couple to continue intimacy without the biological consequences. But sterilization at the beginning of marriage indicates that the couple does not intend to procreate. The faith community surely ought to counsel the couple to consider carefully their decision not to have a child unless there are strong personal health reasons for doing so.

The issue of forced sterilization on criminals, psychopaths, and persons with strong genetic faults raises an entirely different question. At the present time neither the church nor the society at large recognizes the sexual situation of such persons. Certainly sterilization ought not to be forced on anyone, except in rare cases. The church should counsel and advocate the normalcy of sexual relationships for all people, insofar as that is humanly possible.

The time of conception frequently has been defined as the point at which the sperm penetrates the egg. From a faith perspective, this type of scientific explanation will not suffice. The conception of a child depends as much on the mutual desire of the parents as it does on the union of sperm and egg. For the faith community, conception or procreation depends primarily on the attraction of a woman and a man to each other and their wish to create a loving environment into which a child can be born. The willingness and desire to have a child may not coincide at all with the actual moment of fertilization. But to ignore the faith perception of conception is to ignore much of the moral nature of birth. To put it bluntly, anything which prevents the willing parents from reaching fertilization could be considered wrong. Anything which facilitates the reaching of that inception would be considered morally appropriate.

Artificial Insemination

Because by means of artificial insemination a child can be conceived without the act of love, there are some religious groups
which prohibit it. Yet the desire to procreate, the acts of sexual
intimacy, and the fertilization of the egg are not necessarily
simultaneous. Once there is a desire to create a child, from the
covenant perspective there is no reason, within the limits of
medical safety, for the couple not to use drugs or mechanical
means to increase the possibility of fertilization. For some few
couples, there can be insemination outside the womb (*in
vitro*). The eventuality of *in vitro* fertilization does place the
issue of intimacy in its sharpest focus. From a covenant
standpoint, the desire of the couple to have a child determines
the morality of the way in which that is accomplished.

Surrogate Motherhood

In this last few years another ethical issue has arisen. At the
time of this writing, about five hundred children have been
born from surrogate mothers. The use of one mother to
create a child for another has an ancient precedent. In the pat-
riarchal narrative of Genesis surrogate motherhood plays a
very important role. Abraham and Sarah were promised a
child, one who would be a means of blessing the nations
(Genesis 15:4). The promised child did not come so Hagar
was utilized as a surrogate mother. Though Hagar's son,
Ishmael, was not accepted as the promised child, neither he
nor the practice was condemned. Likewise when Jacob's
beloved Rachel could not bear children, her maid Bilhah was
used to raise up children for her. The practice is not mentioned again in the biblical narrative. Other barren women,
such as the mother of Samson or Hannah, the mother of
Samuel, are praised for their receptivity and faith.

The covenant nature of life includes both biological and
relational reality. While a childless couple may use any avail-

able means to facilitate pregnancy, the use of an egg or sperm from another person must be considered quite another issue. From a covenant perspective a mother cannot easily part from her baby even though the father has not made a faith covenant with her. Likewise, from a covenant perspective, it seems unlikely that a child would come to adulthood without deep concern for her or his biological birth. The case of Baby M indicates the difficulty. At the end of the pregnancy the mother recognized that the child was hers and sued to keep it (see the Case Study at the end of this chapter). The damage of trying to determine who the parents of a child are, either at time of birth or later in life, appears to outweigh the parents' satisfaction of creating a child by one parent when both cannot be involved.

Even though there are only a few such cases, the issue of surrogate motherhood has received wide attention. A survey of 65 bills in 26 states and the District of Columbia in the *Chicago Tribune* indicated that 21 would allow surrogacy, 22 would prohibit, 2 would attempt to stop the exchange of money, and 20 asked for further study.

Sperm Banks

Even though the issue of surrogate motherhood attracts more legal and ethical attention, it must be noted that artificial insemination by a donor constitutes the same problem. That is, a man has "sold" his fatherhood to a couple who cannot conceive. In the case of surrogate motherhood the pregnancy is public and the mother's womb is the locus for prenatal care. But the issue of artificial insemination by a donor is the same. Even though anonymity for the surrogate father can usually be maintained, still children often seek their biological father and in some cases the biological father has sought visiting privileges.

In my view, conception should be considered as much covenantal as biological; still there is an interrelationship between biology and covenant which cannot be ignored.

If a couple cannot conceive then adoption, which places both parents on the same plane, would be preferable to the use of a biological substitute for a mother or father.

Abortion

Probably no other issue has more divided Americans than the issue of abortion. Although it would be inappropriate to associate the issue of abortion strictly with feminism, in our time the two have become rather tightly interlocked. The argument that a woman has the right to determine the future of her own body is well grounded in western, Enlightenment, rationalist thought and has brought various courts to agree that abortions may be legalized. Many oppose this trend as anti-family and anti-religion. Whatever else comes out of the issue of the abortion controversy in our day, two things are clear. First, the sexual relationship is a mutual relationship. No man has the right to use the body of a woman or to cause her to be pregnant without her consent. The sexual relationship and the procreative act must be mutual. When it is put that way, the faith community understands that the issue is not strictly what to do with unwanted pregnancy, but what to do with a society where unwanted children can be conceived. By and large this is what is involved in the problem of male abuse of the female body. In that sense, it is correctly understood as a feminist problem.

But, in the second place, the issue is not strictly that of any one individual alone. In covenant theology one cannot speak of the rights of the fetus or the rights of a woman. Justice for both occurs in a social context. The question of abortion would not arise if we did not live in a society where men could take advantage of women or where unwanted conceptions could occur.

As indicated in the section on narrative ethics, we can deal from a covenant perspective with how life should be, and where society is going. But we live in an imperfect world.

There are dangerous and unwanted pregnancies. Knowing there is no covenantal solution to these problems, how shall the faith community respond when they occur?

There are different kinds of unwanted pregnancies, of course. Most obvious are those where some danger is involved. Many Christian groups would agree that when the mother's life is endangered, then an abortion, though understood as not the perfect will of God, nevertheless may be necessary.

Abortion decisions in rape cases are less clear. There has been no covenant relationship between the woman and the man and the child almost always is unwanted. Violence has replaced love. In such cases, immediate termination of the pregnancy may be the best solution. This is particularly true for the mother if "day after" drugs can be developed reliably. But the grace of God moves in mysterious ways. We have no right to say that the fetus must be terminated. The faith community should support the abused woman, regardless of her decision, and encourage society at large to do the same.

The case of illegitimate children presents yet another problem. Though much of the educational world may consider teen-age pregnancies a result of inadequate sex education, it is much more likely that teen-age pregnancies result from family and societal faults. Young people want to have children in order to create relationships for themselves rather than allowing intimate relationships between a father and mother to result in children. Often there is at least some relationship between the father and the mother of the illegitimate baby and the child may be wanted by one parent or the other. In such a case, the destruction of the fetus could violate the covenant ethics we have described. However, a world which contains a large number of children born or raised in single parent situations may perpetuate the family and social faults that led to the problem of illegitimacy in the first place. Yet it is difficult to believe that abortion is the answer to this problem. There may be no solution for this difficult problem other than for the Christian community to state more forthrightly the meaning of covenant and intimate relationships in the act of procreation.

Unplanned Pregnancies

The issues between the pro-life people, those who deny the legitimacy of abortion, and the pro-choice people, those who believe abortion should be an option for the woman, are no sharper than at this point. No system is perfect. The sterilization process is not absolute; no means of contraception provides 100 percent safety; marital or extra-marital relationships almost always have the potential for pregnancy. In these situations, the context of covenant is assumed, but the child may not be wanted. Do the mother and father, or just the mother, have the right to "use extreme contraception" after fertilization has occurred? Or should the couple accept the unplanned child as one of the gifts of the covenant relationship?

Needless to say, the complexities in either direction could be enormous. In contrast to the couple that wanted children and therefore, in a sense, conceived before fertilization, the unplanned child requires conception after fertilization. That undoubtedly happens. One cannot simply define life as the inception of the fetus, nor can one define it as some specific point, such as the second trimester of pregnancy. When the parents and the community know the child, then the child exists. It is extremely difficult to define such a point, though one suspects the outer limits would be four or five months. Normally one would assume that a relationship has been developed much earlier. Can a couple destroy their own procreative efforts without damage to themselves? Probably not. Are there instances when the parents, and society, would be better if the pregnancy were terminated? Yes, probably.

The believers' church understands that it cannot give correct answers to wrong problems. There are not correct answers in the issue of abortion. The church can help redefine the meaning of life so that persons can make decisions in terms of their faith rather than in terms of a biological timeline. The Free Church also considers preventive medicine, if it may be so called, most important in terms of abortion. That is, the faith community will want to work for a society where men do not take advantage of women, and where children are the result of intimacy rather than objects used to create intimacy.

Severely Impaired Children

The problems raised by the birth of severely impaired children have become increasingly complex. The possibility of having a child with some sort of congenital birth defect has always held a fear for parents. In the past, such children died in their early years, so the problem of caring for them was not as great. Severely impaired children often have been institutionalized although some parents have found it meaningful to care for the children in their home. Though the economic, physical, and emotional burdens of keeping such a child can be enormous, many parents believe that the covenantal relationship between parents and an impaired child can be very close. In more recent years medical technology has reached such a point that many children with congenital defects can be saved, although this does not mean that they can be made normal. Strictly speaking, the issue of severely impaired children will be dealt with under genetics (chapter eleven), but without the possibility of genetic engineering, how can the church best deal with a child born with serious physical or mental impairment?

In recent times the Federal government has moved to protect such children. Under the guise of protecting the civil rights of a class of people, the Department of Health and

Human Services has issued directives that the lives of impaired children are to be saved where possible. The courts, however, have determined that parents and doctors do have the right to decide whether heroic measures should be employed to save the life of the child.

From a covenant perspective, it is the quality of relationship that counts, rather than the "biological" quality of the persons involved. The fact that people are deformed, limited, or marginal does not necessarily affect the quality of the relationship. In fact, it often enhances it. Historically, Jews and Christians have always been concerned about marginal people. At the same time, the emphasis upon relationship implies that the Judeo-Christian tradition does not place its weight upon the sacredness of biological life. There can, and ought to be, times when biological life can be sacrificed for the sake of the relationship. Given the limitation of resources in hospitals, the limitation of beds for ill children, and the limitation of good resources for later health care, it does not seem wise to use extraordinary means to save the life of an impaired child. Again, such decisions should be made with the support of the faith community. The decision to use heroic measures would need to take into consideration the relational need of the parents and the community. Obviously, from a covenantal perspective there are times when the expenditure of excessive resources can be worth the effort. If, however, the child receives unusual treatment simply to save biological life or to provide an opportunity for research, then covenantal relationships themselves may be violated.

The issue of birth is a private matter. Someone has said that we come into this world alone, and we leave the world alone. There is much truth to that and the covenantal ethic attempts to deal with it as sharply as possible. Though birth and death are private matters, the faith community offers to the individual the possibility of making a decision in a supportive context. Questions of abortion and defective birth can be carefully dealt with in a faith setting. A support group that is reflective rather than authoritative may be of enormous value in working through issues relating to birth.

Case Study

William and Elizabeth Stern, of New Jersey, were unable to have children. After trying various methods to facilitate conception, they decided to seek a surrogate mother. Mary Beth Whitehead eventually was hired for $10,000 and was artificially inseminated with sperm from Mr. Stern. Mrs. Whitehead gave birth to a child we know as Baby M. However, she broke the legally drawn up contract and sought to keep the baby. The Sterns then sought legal custody of the child. On March 31, 1987, Superior Court Judge Harvey Sorkow, of New Jersey, ruled that the contract between Mary Beth Whitehead and the Sterns was valid. He awarded custody of Baby M to William and Elizabeth Stern. The baby's biological mother has appealed the decision to the New Jersey Supreme Court, and, as of September 1987, the court has agreed to hear the case.

Questions for Discussion:

1. Should William and Elizabeth Stern have sought a surrogate mother as a means of solving their infertility? Why? Why not?

2. What is the relationship between a biological mother and her child? Is it different for a biological father?

3. Is new life more related to the desire for the child than birthing it? Discuss your reasons for your answer.

7

Death in the Covenant Relationship

Just as the nature of life and its beginning is best understood from the point of view of one's covenant formation, so death is understood primarily in terms of the covenant relationships of later life. Death has been variously defined as the stopping of the heart, the cessation of breathing, or the nonfunction of the brain. From the covenant perspective, however, death occurs when there is no longer the possibility of a mutual relationship.

In the Bible any such disruption of the covenant can be called death. Frequently that may be spoken of as sin, iniquity, illness, or death itself. In the Hebrew scriptures sin results in being cut off from the land of the living (Psalm 52:5). From the faith perspective, such alienation is tantamount to being cast from the presence of God (Psalm 51:11). In the New Testament, Ananias and Sapphira die at the feet of the Apostle Peter because they have falsified their finances to the faith community. Likewise, according to Paul, there are people who are sick and dying at Corinth because they have failed to perceive the body of Christ. Their failure was evident by the fact that they had not shared mutually with the poor in the Love Feast (1 Corinthians 11).

In recent studies of death and dying, it has become clear that separation from significant relationships accompanies the process of death. Given a sufficient period of time, most people will limit primary relationships to friends and family. The next step is to relate only to the family at large. The last stage of covenant dissolution is to close off all but the immediate family or significant others. After that, the dying person becomes inaccessible to everyone. If we follow our covenant understanding of life and death, then this last withdrawal should be defined by the faith community as the stage of death.

The covenant perception of death can accompany the biological, but not necessarily. In fact, the process of death just described probably occurs before a person actually dies biologically. The importance of this cannot be overestimated. When a person has died covenantally, the saving of that person's biological life does not seem true to faith. Yet much of medicine, and even much of theology, assumes the sacredness of biological life. Consequently, health care people are accustomed to saving the biological life long after the person has died relationally, or theologically.

From the point of view of the Christian faith community, the resurrection of the person occurs when these covenant relationships are restored in a redeemed state. Normally the resurrection occurs when family, friends, and wider community meet after the biological death. There, at a funeral or memorial, the loved one is mourned and then the community reestablishes itself with powerful and happy memories of the one who has died. Formation, in this sense, continues. The dead live on in the formation process. In most cultures a meal of re-formation takes place. In many cultures the meal may continue on an annual basis. Only the modern, individualistic, western societies have taken lightly the normal process of death and the gift of resurrection.

This observation has an important effect on the practice of health care for the terminally ill or elderly. Those with a covenantal understanding of death and resurrection know that death occurs when the person loses contact with the basic community, and resurrection occurs when the basic community reestablishes contact without the physical presence of the individual. From the point of view of the faith community, interference with this process has dire results. From the perspective of a believers' church ethicist, such interference is morally wrong. Needless to say, in cases of fatal accidents the dying person is robbed of the opportunity of moving through covenantal death. The attentions of the faith community will need to be turned to the survivors. Likewise, those who cannot or will not, for psychological reasons, respond to covenant relationships also present a special problem.

But when the issue involves the terminally ill, then health care techniques ought not to interfere with the natural process of death and resurrection. Placing terminally ill people in social isolation or in other demeaning and inhumane situations destroys the normal process of death. The church should support whatever measures that would make it possible for the terminally ill and those surrounding her or him to experience death and resurrection.

Heroic Measures

For the most part, extraordinary measures for the terminally ill are based on the assumption that life is sacred. The faith community, with a covenantal view of death, ought to assess those heroic measures which often interfere with the normal process of dying. The family and the support community should resist the temptation to take extraordinary life-saving measures unless there are intervening considerations. The best method to accomplish this is for the family, representatives from the church, and the individual to agree ahead of time about such measures. Increasingly, health care teams honor such agreements. The faith community can also seek prior arrangements with local hospitals. Many hospitals, health care systems, and hospices are willing to allow a representative group of friends and medical people to make decisions about when to use extraordinary measures. Even if the individual has not made a written directive, it may be possible in the future for committees to deal with the issue of death from both a theological and a physical standpoint.

There are a number of arguments involved here. Frequently it is argued that one never knows when resuscitated life will be possible. If the support community asks that extraordinary measures not be used, could such measures have saved the patient? Actually, a person who has died relationally and then has been resuscitated biologically may not be accepted as if the death had never occurred. In other words, persons whose community has accepted their death ought to be allowed to die. The chances of a satisfactory outcome probably do not outweigh the heroic efforts to forestall death and the inappropriate use of health care resources.

How are extraordinary measures defined? For example, are food and water extraordinary? Logically, one would answer that question in the negative. However, many persons are kept alive for months, even years, simply on intravenous feeding. There are many people who do not welcome even that much intervention. Once the process is started, it becomes increasingly difficult to "pull the plug." While one could argue that food and water are not extraordinary measures, what about the use of long-term care facilities? The family along with the faith community will need to make these kinds of decisions on an individual basis.

Euthanasia

Few issues plague the Judeo-Christian conscience more than euthanasia or "mercy killing." The majority of euthanasia cases have probably been dealt with when we say that no heroic means should be used (unless there is reason to suppose that theological death has not occurred). By this we mean that the maintenance of biological life for those who are relationally dead has no basis in the Christian faith. Much more difficult are those instances when the loved one is in extreme pain or has suffered a severely handicapping accident. By and large, the answer to this problem for the faith community would parallel that of birth. As was said about birth, when the community, particularly the mother, can form a relationship with the fetus, then abortion is a very questionable procedure. The same is true of mercy killing. As long as a person has a relationship with others, then euthanasia is a dubious procedure. The process of slow death often is the most significant route for theological death. Relationships can be worked out, sin forgiven, and alienation reconciled. The process of death may be frightening, but it is also highly significant for the covenant community. To rob a person and the community of this process by euthanasia could be a serious wrong.

Suicide

Accurate statistics are not available, but almost everyone agrees that suicide is much more prevalent than would seem apparent. Frequently suicide is an attempt to hurt another individual. The covenant community understands that some persons will injure themselves in order to hurt another person. It is understood, too, that the absence, especially the final absence, of a covenantally-related person means some form of death to everyone involved. The loss of those who have helped to develop one's formation is very real. Sometimes alienation can become so strong that a person is tempted to take that covenant relationship away from another person. Presumably, that is the source of an angry suicide. Usually those types of suicides make themselves known. Unless the intent is somehow apparent, the suicide has no value.

Much more prevalent are the intentions of individuals who want to prevent difficulties for their loved ones, or pain for themselves, by terminating their life in some fashion. This is especially true for older people. The National Center for Health Statistics notes in 1983 a suicide rate of 19.3 per 100,000 for persons over 65, compared to 12.1 for all ages. Some experts project that many traffic accidents are such suicides. Since suicides occur as a protection of self, kindness or love to others, or as a means of protecting pension and insurance plans, often they are undetectable as suicides. Though there may be a laudatory sense in such decision making, the same thing must be said here as has been said about euthanasia. To take one's life before the primary community and the faith community have had time to work through the meaning of death robs everyone of the opportunity to die with a sense of fulfillment.

Hospices

As Christian groups have become more aware of relational issues in regard to dying, they have turned to additional forms of care for the terminally ill. Understandably, the best caregiving place for the terminally ill often is the home. Home care is becoming increasingly popular. However, home care often is impossible because of the nature of the home and the nature of the care required. As a consequence, the faith community should encourage support of the hospice movement which was developed in order to allow persons to deal with their terminal illness in a context of support and acceptance. Hospices allow for the family to be present with the patient more than in other health care giving situations. Those who believe in covenant health care ethics will join with like-minded persons to create hospices in all areas of the country.

The issue of "what covenant?" becomes important at this point. It should not be assumed that the covenant of origin, the family, is actually the closest relationship. Many people find that their peers are closer to them than their family. In this case, the retirement home and its adjacent nursing home, may offer the best alternative. It can still be argued, however, that all too many nursing homes have not been designed to allow for the more home-like atmosphere of the hospice. The faith community needs to influence the design and execution of plans and procedures for such institutions (private institutions, hospitals, nursing homes, and private homes) so that the terminally ill are given the maximum covenant possibility until the time of death.

Organ Transplant

As we have already seen, the Christian understanding of resurrection primarily involves a loving relationship within the covenant group of the deceased. This provides a continued role for the departed dead in the ongoing formation process of the faith community. That covenant community, called the Body, or the Body of Christ, is the locus of resurrection of individuals. In the New Testament, that new life is referred to as "resurrection from among dead ones," or, "resurrection of the body." The understanding that resurrection involves the physical components, or flesh, of an individual does not occur in the New Testament. In fact, it did not come into play until after the fourth century. Often it has been pointed out that early persecutors of Christianity thought they might dissuade believers from resistance and martyrdom by destroying their bodies after death. The plan did not work, and there were even more martyrs and resistance. This is a clear indication that the early Christians were not deterred by the knowledge that their physical bodies might be dismembered or destroyed. They understood that "resurrection of the body" involved their relationship with the faith community.

Christians, then, have no reason to avoid organ transplants. The possibility of giving life to another person through donation of organs at death, or even prior to death, seems most appropriate. In the late 1980's, however, a method for the just distribution of available organs is not apparent. Transplant operations are very expensive, and the availability of organs for such transplants is quite limited. There is as yet no equitable way to deal with this issue. Given current conditions, there may never be a just way of deciding who receives transplants and who does not. As long as that is true, it cannot be said unequivocally that Christians should support the current interest in transplants. However, there is no Judeo-Christian reason why one should avoid making a living will or offering one's organs for transplant.

In the fall of 1987 surgeons in Mexico City transplanted brain tissue from a nonviable fetus into the brains of two men suffering from Parkinson's disease. Their formal report, made early in 1988, indicated a measurable improvement on the part of the two patients. The ethical issues were immediately apparent. While there is no objection to the use of the organs of a "dead" fetus for transplants, the faith community must object to the vindication of abortion as a means of obtaining fetal organs or tissue. Even more sinister would be the conception of a fetus for the purpose of obtaining such life-giving material.

Case Study

A young man is badly injured when a leaking propane gas line explodes, an accident in which his father is killed. He has second- and third-degree burns over 68 percent of his body; his eyes, ears, and most of his face are burned away. After many months of skin grafts, his hands have been amputated, he is susceptible to infections, and he has to be bathed daily in a special tank. Although he accepts treatment, he says he wants to die. Eventually he refuses further treatment and insists on going home—a move that would mean sure and early death. His mother opposes his decision, and a psychiatrist agrees to see him, after getting the impression that he is irrational and depressed. Perhaps he should be declared incompetent so that a legal guardian can authorize treatment. Instead, the psychiatrist finds the young man to be bright, coherent, logical, and articulate—anything but incompetent. He says, "I do not want to go on as a blind and crippled person." He wants his attorney to have him released from the hospital, by court order if necessary. (Taken from *Hard Choices*, p. 21)

Questions for Discussion:

1. The young man can give informed consent. Should he be allowed to determine whether he lives or not?

2. In terms of a covenant faith when will the young man die?

3. Even if you are not willing for a "physician to administer aid in dying," under what circumstances would you allow the natural death which would result if treatments were no longer offered or accepted?

8

The Distribution of Health Resources

Though justice is an end-time expectation, and though Christians will work for final justice, justice deals primarily with life between the beginning and the end. Decisions should be made in terms of creation and end time, but we live in a world which lies somewhere between. It is in such a world where we must act ethically. Consequently the issue of justice becomes very important.

As has been noted, the people of the covenant do not recognize the modern dichotomy between individual and community. Much of western civilization, and particularly the American sense of justice, depends upon an individualistic perception. The United States Constitution protects the rights of individuals, particularly with reference to property. When Americans think of medical ethics, they frequently think in terms of those rights. This leads many people to somewhat different conclusions about medical ethics than that which has been presented in this discussion. The other great system of justice comes from Marxism. In socialist countries, the good of the whole people (the "workers") takes priority over the rights of the individual. This is the basis of justice, for example, in the USSR. Consequently, United States foreign policy has consistently attacked the Soviet Union on human rights issues. Soviet officials often fail to understand this criticism. It is because these two super-states function out of differing views of justice.

The life of the covenant community does not operate with either a Marxist or democratic individualist sense of justice. Since our understanding of God is nearly synonymous with our understanding of the corporate total, the covenant community must be concerned about the good of the whole. This seems to lean toward a socialist model. However, because each individual is formed through the corporate total, then the "justice" of the individual represents the justice of the whole. While it is true that the faith community does not act to protect the rights of individuals *per se*, nevertheless injustice to one individual condemns the whole social structure. In this context, one does not speak of rights so much as corporate conscience.

Under moral pressure a democratic society will work to increase the rights of each citizen. Socialist countries will strive to increase the quality of corporate life. The covenant community, under that same moral pressure, will try to raise the consciousness of all members of society so that each person can become a legitimate participant in the total life. That sense of justice (Hebrew: *mishpat*) is so strong that it can override almost everything else. The interesting case of Tamar in Genesis 38 shows such an overriding sense of justice. Tamar had a right to levirate marriage (a widow's right to a family from her dead husband's brothers) from the sons of Judah. But because of fear, Judah refused to give her yet another son. Consequently the family of Tamar, and even the nature of the society, was threatened. Tamar took things into her own hands. She acted as a prostitute and enticed Judah into the levirate marriage. Even though her action was immoral, it accomplished justice. Judah recognized that fact and overlooked her immorality. The story of Tamar states justice so powerfully that she is even mentioned in the genealogy of Jesus.

When there were poor in the land and orphans or widows were not being treated with mutuality, the prophets tried to raise the consciousness of the society. They were horrified that people with wealth could stand before God and worship when they lived in a society without justice. Such behavior seemed a lie to the prophets. Recognition of the whole requires a consciousness of the corporate nature of society. In this sense, the Judeo-Christian awareness of persons in society differs radically from modern western as well as socialist points of view.

Historically, then, the church has insisted on care for persons on the fringe, the poor, the disabled, the handicapped, the aged, and others who appear marginalized. In fact, a society is measured by the way in which it cares for those who are not equal to the norm in terms of skill or merit. The Hebrew scriptures speak of God's everlasting love (*chesed*) for such persons. In the New Testament, the norm is *agape* love, or self-giving love. We are all marginal except for the grace of God. In self-giving love, the one who gives to the marginalized understands that it should result in a mutual relationship. This is the meaning of Jesus Christ on the cross. The action of God in Christ enables mutuality within the faith community, the Body of Christ. Historians point out that Christianity eventually combined *agape* with other forms of love in the ancient world, so that we finally ended up with love which reforms (Latin: *caritas*). We know this love as charity or philanthropy. Covenant communities based on a New Testament model would prefer, however, to see a love which creates mutuality, rather than a love which tries to reform the other person. In our day, the latter is described frequently as paternalism.

Justice in Health Care

Though there may be many persons who prefer a *laissez-faire* approach to health care without governmental direction, most would recognize that such an approach to medicine means that the wealthy receive excellent care while the poor do not. Not only has the Judeo-Christian tradition understood this, but American society, as well as many others, has recognized the obligation of the state to the indigent and the elderly.

Some persons argue that distribution of health resources ought to be equal, except for circumstances when some key people ought to have access to additional health resources. The logic of this position hardly can be denied. Advocates of this ethic would argue that in the case of the lifeboat analogy mentioned earlier (see chapter four), the survivors in the boat ought to make sure that the navigator stays alive and alert. Yet, the Judeo-Christian faith, by and large, does not give that much credence to specialization and knowledge. While the faith community does not want to be ignorant or obtuse, it believes that the Holy Spirit creates within the community those functions necessary for its own life and purpose.

Others believe that health care resources ought to be allocated according to merit. Additional medical resources should be given to people for their contribution to society not because of their wealth or importance. This is surely one of the more painful aspects of American health care ethics. There are unquestionably differences in terms of what individuals contribute to society. Perhaps it is the relative newness of American society, but the problem of forming a composite society still haunts us. We want an egalitarian society. Yet, there are persons who "do not pull their weight" in an industrialized society. As we have seen in the biblical covenant story, however, the sense of mutual community does not support the granting of additional resources for persons of merit. Indeed, the Bible does not recognize that some have merit while others do not. The prophet Nathan made it clear to David that he had no right to the wife of Uriah. In the same way the prophet Elijah made it clear to King Ahab that he had no right to the vineyard of Naboth.

Because of the complexities of resources distribution today, many ethicists say that justice can only be done when access to health care resources depends on chance. Unless there are extraordinary reasons, persons will be given access to limited resources according to first-come, first-served, or according to chance. Most hospitals allowed to do transplants now operate according to the order of application. When an organ becomes available for transplant, the next person on the list has an opportunity to receive it.

American society has been troubled in recent years by media appeals for transplant resources. The appearance of a small child on television who needs a heart or liver puts that child at the top of the list. It is difficult for Christians to argue that such a child should take a rightful position at a lower place in the order. It would be appropriate, though, for Christian groups to argue for chance, rather than to allow some group, such as the media, to determine who will get the resources. A lottery system has approximately the same effect, except that it may be even more of a random chance. In the Hebrew scriptures, casting lots was used with some degree of frequency in order to prevent the community from giving preference to someone with merit or position. For example, according to one narrative Saul was elected king through lot (1 Samuel 10:20–24). In the New Testament Matthias was elected an apostle by lot (Acts 1:26). A chance or lot, like the Year of Jubilee (Leviticus 25) in which property was to be returned, reminds us that all of us are marginal and have no claim on life except as a gift of God (1 Corinthians 1:26–31).

Finally, Christians in particular would argue that people should receive resources according to need. Operating out of the same sense of *agape* found in the New Testament, we can see that New Testament figures were self-giving to those in need. In Acts 3, as John and Peter were walking in the temple area, they met a lame man who was begging. Admitting they had no money, they would give everything they could.

What they had to give was the healing of the man born lame. Giving even to the point of self-destruction is looked upon as a virtue in most of the New Testament. Jesus highly praised the widow who gave all that she had. It must be stated, however, that while giving of self in the extreme may be laudable, it can be destructive to the person who is the recipient. The purpose of giving is not simply charity, but a means of restoring the mutuality of the individual in the community. It should function to restore identity and purpose for the one who receives it. Restoration to mutuality better reflects the biblical sense of justice than the kinds of altruism and good will that is found often in the modern world.

Just as health results from forgiveness in the community and our return to it, so also covenant justice is the process of that restoration. This means that any other principle of justice will eventually fail. For example, the people of the ancient Near East often lived by *lex talionis* (the law of retaliation in which the punishment fits the crime). This principle may have been a great deterrent, but Jesus, in the Sermon on the Mount (Matthew 5:38–39), noted that the law of retaliation would not bring about reconciliation. This can be said about any type of general law or principle.

It is for this reason that the church, the community of Jesus, should become deeply involved in health care ethics. In the public realm many health care decisions will be made on the basis of merit or perhaps wealth. A congregational health care committee can advocate a health care system which allows the best for each person. But if one principle must be followed, then that principle should be a lottery. By using a lottery, no one presumes to know why a certain action is taken. It is with the providence of God. Even though reconciliation and justice may not be accomplished, at least they are not set askew.

Case Study

In June of 1986, Baby Jesse was brought to the Loma Linda hospital in California with a failing heart where it was determined that a heart transplant was the only possibility for the survival of the baby. Some persons have estimated that as many as 400 hearts are needed for infants each year and perhaps five become available at the right time. Hospitals, therefore, feel the burden of making a responsible selection.

Selection is usually done in two stages. The first stage is to reduce the number of potential recipients by using criteria such as the following: general health, probability of success, continuing care after the operation, the ability of the baby's caretakers to provide. When the potential recipients have been reduced to the most worthy, then the second-stage selection is made. The second stage is usually a matter of chance, such as first-come, first-served.

Baby Jesse's mother was a teenager, unmarried and with few financial resources. The father was a man in his twenties. The hospital determined that under the circumstances the probability of continuing good care was low enough that Baby Jesse ought not be considered a potential recipient of a heart.

It should also be noted that medical specialists do not know how long infants with heart transplants will survive. Too few such operations have been performed to have accumulated much experience. The hope is that recipients can survive several years or even several decades. Furthermore, a person with a heart transplant must have a biopsy performed regularly, twice a year or more for life, to determine whether the heart is being rejected. Care for such a child is much more than abnormal, and of course expense is considerably greater.

When it became public information that Baby Jesse was not to be included as a potential recipient of a heart, a public protest developed. During that time the grandparents indicated that they would be willing to assume responsibility for the care of the infant. Because of the grandparents' decision, the hospital decided to include Baby Jesse among potential recipients. The national publicity caught the attention of a parent in the Midwest whose infant was brain dead. This parent offered the heart of the brain dead child to Baby Jesse and the transplant was performed.

Questions for Discussion:

1. Do you agree with the hospital that exceptional measures (like a heart transplant) should not be used if an infant lacks a caring, viable community context? Or do you consider all life sacred?

2. Should the transplant have been a matter of chance (lottery) regardless of the merits of the case? How would you feel about the lottery if you needed a transplant?

3. Should public opinion and the media be allowed to determine who receives medical resources? How would you control or prevent public appeals?

9

Lifestyle and Health

For the most part, the biblical narrative and covenant theology does not recognize a purely individual lifestyle. Since the individual is a part of the community and has resulted from the formation of the community, then any ethic, however individualistic it might look, actually comes from and affects that community. Individuals perform moral acts. Yet it is extremely difficult to think of any moral action or concern which does not affect, in some way, the community of which a person is a part.

Nevertheless, there are some health decisions today that western society considers primarily individual lifestyle decisions. The believers' churches, however, have long held that such lifestyle issues are social concerns and ought to be dealt with corporately. There are at least three aspects of lifestyle which are very important to issues of medical ethics. These are personal health care, chemical dependency, and sexual relationships.

Personal Health Standards

The American culture is flooded with all manner and methods for keeping healthy. The reason for so many possibilities points to a major concern for health ethics. The

American people have failed to live in such a way as to preserve the health they should have. At least two of the top ten killers in America, strokes and heart attacks, are due to diet and health standards. For the faith community the issue is that of the simple life. The New Testament calls for disciples of Jesus to live on a day-to-day basis. The disciple recognizes that the birds and the flowers are not concerned for tomorrow. In 1 Corinthians 7 Paul says that Christians are to live in a state of tension with the end time. They are to continue in this life, but they are not to regard this life as ultimate reality. The Christian doctrine of the simple life is, finally, an end-time way of thinking. It enables us to be free of the destructive powers of this age.

The decision to live simply may appear to be an individual decision, but that is not true. One does not enter the Kingdom of God alone; it takes a *community* of believers to develop the *qualities* of God's new reign. The new community of God's Kingdom helps the individual both in terms of correct choices as well as support in those choices. Each local congregation should have some persons who are able to make available the best advice for diets, exercise, and good health habits. While one group in the church should deal with advice and education, another group should be of a caring and supportive nature. Buying groups such as food cooperatives could help locate and distribute nutritional foods. It is generally agreed that most people who are alcoholic or overweight need something like Alcoholics Anonymous or Weight Watchers to help them understand their problem and then continue to live in their new state of freedom. If the local faith community cannot develop such groups, then it would do well to cooperate with other groups to accomplish the aims for a simpler, healthier lifestyle.

Chemical Dependency

The misuse of drugs may at first seem to be a simple matter;

however, it is not. From the perspective of the faith community there are two negative elements in drug abuse. The first is a faith problem and the second a medical problem. The human personality or *psyche* develops from interaction in the basic community. The use of certain drugs becomes a synthetic way of altering those relationships. Writers in health ethics normally refer to the use of drugs as an invasion of privacy, but the covenant Christian considers it an invasion of social relationships. Often drugs are used because of unsatisfactory social relationships. That is, a person uses drugs in order to make social adjustments. This means the problems of the social fabric itself are not addressed. Included in such a list of drugs taken for this purpose are nicotine, alcohol, tranquilizers, sleeping medications, marijuana, hallucinatory chemicals, and perhaps some foods such as chocolate and caffeine beverages.

In the view of the faith community use of drugs parallels the problem of false witness. False witness gives a wrong perspective on the community and the process of justice. It does not enable the community to deal effectively with its own problems. The use of chemicals to alter one's behavior patterns creates a false sense of identity and security. But the combination of alienation from the faith community and the misuse of drugs creates dangerous health problems in American society. The following drugs illustrate this point.

1. *Nicotine:* The relationship of nicotine to lung cancer has been clearly demonstrated. In 1971 US Surgeon General Luther Terry forbade radio and TV advertisement for cigarettes, forced the tobacco industry to publish a warning message on cigarette packages, and to acknowledge the dangers inherent in the use of tobacco. Since 1971 adults have cut back appreciably, but 53,000,000 Americans still use tobacco in some form. However, youth have not only ignored the warning, but have significantly increased their use of the drug. One example is the statistic that indicates that

ten times the number of twelve-year-old girls smoke cigarettes today than prior to 1971.

As a consequence, nicotine still ranks as one of the major health hazards in America. For many older adults, the use of nicotine has appeared to be an individual choice. Increasingly, that is less true. Medical research has shown that para-nicotine usage is nearly as serious as the use of nicotine itself. That is, people who are continually in the presence of smokers also have a higher chance of lung cancer. Consequently, the mood of the American lawmakers at the moment is toward the exclusion of smoking in public places and in the work place as well. One company, for example, has set a policy that people who smoke will not be hired, and their employees who smoke will be offered treatment to help them quit. More and more, smoking is being banned from public transportation and in public buildings.

The question of individual right and community responsibility looms high in this instance. For many, smoking is an individual choice and society should not invade the privacy of the individual. But, it is increasingly apparent that smoking shortens both the life of those who smoke and those who breathe second-hand smoke. Not only is life shortened, but valuable health resources are used to care for such persons.

As in weight watching and alcoholism, the faith community should find ways of supporting persons who wish to stop using nicotine. Simultaneously, the faith community should apply no less than gentle pressure to ban the use of tobacco in public places.

2.*Alcohol:* Historically speaking, the social or medical use of beverage alcohol has not been a problem for the believers' churches, although many have taken strong temperance positions. Though drunkenness is condemned in the Bible (1 Corinthians 6), the use of wine generally is not. In fact, in 1 Timothy, absence from the use of wine is seen as a gnostic (spiritualistic) misunderstanding of creation.

However, today's urban and industrial society is not the same as that of ancient Palestine. There are problems with alcohol today that apparently were minor in those days. Social and moderate drinking, to say nothing of alcoholism, make it a serious ethical problem. There are about 60,000 deaths a year in the United States due to automobile accidents as well as the even larger number of injuries. A vast number of these accidents are alcohol-related, many of which are related to teenage drinking. Given the number of deaths and injuries, and the medical resources that are used to care for them, one would expect society to be as concerned with the drinking driver as with cancer. This is not the case. The faith community needs to put considerable effort into the control of alcohol in society.

At the same time, certain persons are trapped by the disease of alcoholism. It is still not medically clear whether this entrapment—alcoholism—has a genetic basis or results from habit-forming use. Currently, it is generally assumed that alcoholism is an inherited problem. The disease creates a certain type of personality with alcoholic tendencies, whether alcohol itself becomes involved or not. Inherited or habit, alcoholism has reached serious proportions in modern society. Not only does it waste lives and destroy families, but it also creates diet and lifestyle problems that can require hospitalization.

The church can do a great deal to support persons who are attempting to stay away from the use of alcohol, particularly those who may be dependent types. The faith community needs to understand that this is not easy, because acceptance of the alcoholic personality may not be therapeutic. A program of both discipline and care must be exercised. Many people in the faith community believe that some form of treatment like Alcoholics Anonymous may be the only way to deal effectively with the alcoholic-type personality. The church will want to support such efforts, both within the Judeo-Christian tradition and outside it.

3. *Marijuana, Uppers, and Downers:* The final word has not been written on mood-altering drugs. They appear to be habit-forming. But the extent to which such drugs might be involved in accidents or serious health problems is not clear. It is not presently believed by the medical community that these drugs are as serious as alcohol. The same objections can be raised to mood-altering drugs as any type of chemical dependency. Use of these drugs avoids the issue of the social relationship. A more important consideration, however, is that the use of mood-altering drugs can lead to the use of stronger, hallucinatory drugs. Again, whether this is primarily a personality-relational issue is not absolutely clear. At this time the best approach for the church is to support efforts, particularly those in the media and public education, which encourage persons to stay away from such drugs altogether. At the same time, there should be within the faith community, the pastor or some other caregiver, who can counsel or refer for such counseling persons who are involved in using mood-altering drugs.

4. *Hallucinatory Drugs:* Hard drugs, such as heroin, cocaine, and crack, are both dangerous to persons and destructive of society. The heaviest use of hard drugs comes from those parts of society that are the most alienated. They provide a sense of escape, but at a terrible price. The problem of hallucinatory drugs is so pervasive in our society that the faith community has no choice but to operate on at least three levels. First, it must assist those forces which would prevent the availability of such drugs to persons who are potential users. Second, professionals in health care should set up detoxification programs. Third, many denominations and some local congregations either have developed or have joined with local groups or agencies to help people break the drug habit.

As with the issue of abortion, the real issue with hard drugs is a society in which their use is viewed as a way of dealing with problems. The end-time goal of the faith community should be to create a society in which hallucinatory drugs are not functional. Chief among these problems would be issues of alienation, unemployment, ghettoization, and abuse of persons. A major concern of the faith community anywhere, but especially in inner city situations, should be to allow all persons to find mutual significance in their life with others.

Medicinal Use of Drugs

Not all drug abuse, however, is voluntary or forced alteration of the individual psyche in order to deal with the social structure. In contrast to drugs used for social purposes are those drugs prescribed by physicians to alter personality abnormalities. As more and more about behavior patterns and genetics is understood, it appears likely that chemical means of altering behavior will become more prevalent. At the present time there are at least two well-known character disorders that can be somewhat controlled by chemical means. Schizophrenia is a mental illness characterized by psychotic thinking, delusions of persecution or even grandeur, speaking in a disorganized way, hallucinations, and a false perception of reality. Cures for schizophrenia are not easily found, but major tranquilizers like phenothiazine (Praxiline) have proven to be effective in the treatment of the serious psychological disorders that occur in schizophrenia.

Another disorder, hyperactivity or hyperkinesis, is particularly found among children. The hyperkinetic child is restless, moody, irritable, and impulsive. These children cannot concentrate in school, become a problem in the classroom, and do not learn properly. Two drugs, methylphenidate (Ritalin) and amphetamine (Desidrin), have the affect of a stimulant in most people. But with hyperactive children, these drugs have the opposite affect. Generally, children taking either one of these drugs will be able to concentrate better and exhibit more controlled classroom behavior.

At first glance, it would appear that, given proper precautions regarding side-effects, drugs that enable persons to function better in society should be affirmed by the faith community. The believers' churches should review carefully the circumstances for the use of such drugs. There are several problems. Consider, for example, that most ethicists are concerned about the rights of the individual. To what extent do we allow physicians and psychologists to invade the individual personality? Similarly, most of us would reject the right of department stores or the advertising industry to influence buying through subconscious or subliminal advertising messages. Would we resist health care professionals who might use subliminal techniques to control smoking or obesity? Could the excessive violence of American society be controlled by constant patterns of subconscious communication?

At another level, the faith community is more concerned about the formation process than about individual rights. Are "good drugs" used to help control character disorders, or are they part of a cure? Are not these drugs or subliminal suggestions simply ways to help the individual adjust to a society which itself has produced the aberrant person? Are not society and the church avoiding the real health issue through the use of behavior modification drugs, and even through some forms of therapy? While these questions are complex, the believers' church can assume the chemical invasion of an individual's personality, and therefore of the formative community, may be as destructive to society as the problem it strives to correct.

Problems Related to Sexual Intimacy

In the biblical world the formation of persons and their identity is deeply tied to intimacy. Good physical and mental health depends on intimacy. Because the primary unit, the family, is so intimate, personal identity is rooted in the familial process of development and growth. In the New Testament particularly, that intimacy is protected in marriage by the warning that the intimate relationship cannot be superceded by yet another relationship (remarriage after divorce) or by other intimacies. For that reason, idolatry and adultery are closely aligned in biblical thought (see Hosea 1-2). The words of Jesus are particularly powerful at this point. In the Gospel of Mark passage (10:2-12), divorce is considered impossible. If, for any reason, there is divorce and remarriage, then adultery is committed. In Matthew, this expectation is stated so strongly that followers are encouraged not to remarry under any circumstances. The disciples are aghast at the difficult nature of Jesus' teaching on divorce. The same concern may be seen in Paul's instructions to the Corinthians (1 Cor. 7:1-24) where it is clear that a second marriage may be permitted. But even then remarriage is a concession. These scriptural passages suggest that the Judeo-Christian tradition has a very strong sense of the permanence of intimacy.

This regard for the power and joy of intimacy creates a very important concern for right relationships. Yet a difficulty occurs when it comes to sexually oriented health problems within marriage, such as impotency, frigidity, sexual identity, fertility, and sexually transmitted diseases. While being compassionate for those who experience sexually oriented problems, the faith community must call for a lifestyle where intimacy does not result in poor physical and emotional health. If the faith community calls for a world which does not know war, rather than calling for a world which is compassionate to warriors; if the faith community calls for a world where women are treated appropriately, rather than developing a massive abortion system; if the faith community calls for a world which does not need drugs, rather than developing massive detoxification clinics; then the faith community here calls for a world where intimacy has its rightful value, rather than primarily addressing the results of the tragic failure of marriage and family life in our society. That concern must be stated first, but it is more than a concern. The educational and social structures of the faith community ought to be oriented strongly toward developing a society where intimacy produces health.

Nevertheless, the failure of the system has given to the world of the late twentieth century some problems of gigantic proportion. Any health care ethic must deal with these problems. In the early 1980s the basic threat was sexually contracted herpes simplex. But by 1985 an entirely new problem arose. The possibility of a pandemic killer sexual disease has frightened the entire world. This disease is AIDS.

Acquired Immune Deficiency Syndrome (AIDS)

AIDS is the result of a virus labeled HIV, Human Immunodeficiency Virus. The virus apparently lives in a number of people, but eventually some people who carry the virus will exhibit the symptoms of AIDS. There is no known cure for AIDS.

The AIDS virus is evident primarily among the homosexual population. Some 73 percent of the diagnosed cases have been practicing homosexuals. Another 16 percent of AIDS patients have used unsanitary hypodermic needles. A few cases (3-4 percent) have occurred in persons who have experienced blood transfusions, trans-placental (mother to fetus) infection, and heterosexual intercourse. AIDS is a worldwide problem. It is particularly rampant in Africa. Some people estimate as many as 10 million people worldwide will have AIDS before the turn of the century. It is not known to what extent HIV is present in American society. Some persons estimate there are 50 carriers of the virus to every person diagnosed as having AIDS. If that is true, then there are approximately one-and-a-half to two million people infected. As of late 1987 the increase in the number of people diagnosed as having contracted AIDS is not quite as dramatic as in 1986. There is sufficient hope in these statistics to indicate that certain patterns of safe sex can restrict the spread of AIDS in the United States. Perhaps warnings regarding the use of needles and drugs, and warnings against homosexual intimacy and heterosexual promiscuity are having an impact.

Even though one may take some comfort in the fact that the AIDS epidemic seems to be slowing down in the United States, still the issue of sexual diseases remains with us. In some respects, the problem of AIDS in our time parallels the problem of leprosy in the New Testament. People with leprosy were considered unclean and, therefore, could not be a part of normal society. Because of the major ways in which AIDS can be transmitted, the majority of the western world considers persons who contract AIDS as "unclean." In the New Testament Jesus did not ignore socially ostracized people with flows of blood or leprosy.

Throughout the course of Christian history concerned people time and time again have been willing to risk their lives to care for people with contagious diseases such as leprosy or tuberculosis. The Christian attitude toward AIDS should undoubtedly be the same, without regard for how the disease is contracted. Though there may be risk, the church will want to respond compassionately to those with AIDS. Currently AIDS patients are a severe drain on the resources of a hospital. In all probability, sanitariums or specialized hospitals will need to be built in order to give special attention to AIDS patients. In terms of the general population, the faith community will want to encourage people to be knowledgeable about AIDS and not to fear or shun persons who have been diagnosed as having AIDS. Rather, the faith community will give assistance to AIDS victims, even if that does involve risk.

Case Study

A West Coast city is one of a number of places in the United

States where the drug Ritalin (methylphenidate) is used to treat learning disabilities in hyperactive schoolchildren. The parents of seventeen grade-school-age children have brought suit to prevent its use from being mandatory. One of the children, Tommy, was given Ritalin after doctors diagnosed his stuttering and behavioral disturbances as due to hyperactivity. Tommy's parents say they were told there would be no side effects; they therefore gave consent for the treatment, hoping he would slow down and be able to concentrate better. As they understood it, the alternative was to place Tommy in a special class. After Tommy began to take the drug under the supervision of the school physician, his parents say, he became irritable, cried a lot, and had tantrums, headaches, and stomach upsets. They have decided not to allow him to take Ritalin any more and claim they would never have consented in the first place if they had been told of its possible side effects and of their own right to refuse treatment. (Taken from *Hard Choices*, p. 15)

Questions for Discussion:

1. From your covenant understanding of health, do you think Tommy should be made educable by means of drugs? When are drugs acceptable for medicinal purposes?

2. If drugs are not the answer for persons like Tommy, what would you suggest?

3. Did the parents of Tommy give "informed consent"? When did they give it? Did they have the moral right to give consent for drugs to be used? Who does?

10

Health and Social Environment

With the rapid increase in world population, the decrease in resources for some parts of the world, the abuse of our environment, and the pollution of atmosphere and water, the faith community must address environmental issues for the improvement of health levels. The story of creation makes it clear that humans are to have dominion over God's gift. Dominion, however, does not mean abuse or rape.

The biblical doctrine of creation made of Judeo-Christianity a scientific civilization. That is, Judeo-Christians have felt free to investigate the created world and to use the creation for their own benefit. In the Hebrew scriptures God clearly uses the created world for divine purposes. In the middle of battle, the sun can stand still or the earth can open up for divine punishment, or the sea can part for a redemptive act. Thus creation serves more as a sister of humanity than its servant. With humanity, nature too has fallen. In anticipation of the end time, creation yearns for wholeness as does the faith community (Romans 8:23).

Jesus healed people of infirmities and diseases and he could also still the waves and command the wind. Paul spoke of the creation "groaning in travail" until the time of redemption (Romans 8:23). The biblical writers do not specifically attach the healing of persons with the healing of the environ‐ment, but both are assumed to be part of God's reign. We can suppose that dominion over the creation also means health and wholeness to both humanity and nature.

Our generation faces more critical environmental prob‐lems than the world of the New Testament. To be sure there were times of severe famines (2 Corinthians 8:2), floods, and earthquakes. Sometime after the biblical period much of the Near East was deforested. Because of climate and diseases half the children born at that time did not reach ten years of age. In reading ancient history, however, it would appear that the mass of human misery occurred because of human avarice and greed, as well as failure of governments to keep the peace. The world was not overpopulated. Chemical pollu‐tion was unknown, although lack of sanitation caused urban epidemics.

The faith community today faces a large number of complex issues in regard to social environment. Denomina‐tions, judicatories, and church agencies must help the local congregation sort through these issues clearly and recom‐mend action both for the local church and for individuals. In this discussion all of the environmental issues and how they might be approached cannot possibly be mentioned. A few examples will suffice.

World Hunger

Food experts do not agree about the causes for the increase in world hunger. The fact of hunger cannot be denied, but the reasons for it are elusive. There are about 500,000,000 malnourished persons in the world. This means that they lack the essential nutrients to live an active life. Many persons assume that the problem is one of distribution. The presence of stockpiles, attempts to decrease production, and the de‐struction of surpluses lead most people to assume that it is the lack of political and economic power necessary to feed the world that is responsible for world hunger. But that is not a sufficient explanation. If all the resources were distributed equally, then everyone in the world would be under-nourished. Or, if all the food in the world were distributed at the level of consumption found in the United States only about one-third of the world would be fed.

For others the real issue is overpopulation (first described by Thomas Robert Malthus). During the great population explosion of Europe (1850–1950) people could move to new territory. One million Europeans left for North America, South America, Oceania, and Siberia. There they appropriated the best resources, causing in some cases a serious depletion of land and water resources. Now the Third World population is exploding and there is no place to expand. This leaves practically no choice but to insist on birth control in Third World countries. So far that effort, though useful, has not halted the growth of world hunger. To the contrary, food consumption relates to population in some way other than a simple increase in numbers. Affluent societies in which there is a surplus of food and sufficient health care undergo a drop in birth rate. The circle is vicious. Over-populated areas apparently will only curb the rate of birth when the standard of living reaches a satisfactory level.

Yet another cause for hunger is the inequity between rich and poor. For most of the world that division has become incredibly sharp. In Latin America 17 percent of the land-owners control 90 percent of the land. Asia has a better distribution: the upper 20 percent own 60 percent of the useful land. In Africa, about three-fourths of the population have access to about 4 percent of the land. A third of the agricultural population of the world has no access to land at all. This severely inappropriate distribution carries with it yet another problem. The poor countries use their land resources for cash export crops not for food to be consumed by the local population. For example, African nations export grains, nuts, and fresh vegetables, yet have the highest incidence of protein-caloric deficiencies among children. Mexico supplies the United States with over half of its supply of several varieties of winter and spring vegetables. Even more glaring is the use of land for exports which have little value in domestic consumption such as coffee, soybeans, tea, and rubber.

Whatever the causes of malnutrition, the health situation cannot be overestimated. While we are concerned for all the people of the earth, we must also acknowledge that poverty deeply affects health in the United States. It is particularly the children who are seriously threatened. In 1985 over 13,000,000 US children were living in poverty. This will increase as lower income people receive even less, and as government assistance for persons in poverty decreases.

In this complex situation the church understands that human redemption includes the "making whole" of nature. As humanity moves closer to the end time so will the created natural order: the land, water, and other resources. As we believe that all humanity and nature will work together, so we believe in God as universality. Anything less must be idolatry. From this sense of universality comes the responsibility for the worldwide community. We call this concern, in faith terms, political theology.

To assist the worldwide community here are some suggestions:

—offer education and information regarding family planning.

—assist "most seriously affected" countries with agricultural development programs;

—lobby to prevent multi-national, agri-business companies from investing in "most seriously affected" countries;

—lobby to prevent United States companies from importing food products from hunger-ridden countries;

—with due caution offer food supplies during severe famine periods.

The relationship of developed countries to the less developed has been one, on the whole, of beneficial patronage. The patron-client mentality set up a system of colonialism which plagues our world today. The developed countries "assist" the "most seriously affected" countries by making investments in them, building their infrastructures (transportation, communication, and so forth), importing from them, and offering them military protection. This system creates a poverty from which there is no escape. At the same time, political independence achieved by former colonies or client states offers little hope. Some countries, having been dependent, simply do not have the leadership and resources to exist alone in the modern world. As a result poverty increases and future health problems multiply. The populace has been set up, so to speak, for such widespread epidemics as the current AIDS crisis. Politically observant Christians have become more and more convinced that developed and less-developed countries must exist in some mutual relationship. This is nowhere more evident than in world mission programs. The parent denomination or agency and the indigenous church must share resources and trained personnel in such a way that allocation decisions are made by a mutual process. Each partner has something to give, and receive. In a similar way the present pattern in international relations must be changed through a mutual sharing and a mutual decision making.

Environmental Pollution

Serious as the problem of world hunger is, pollution of air, land, and water presents the most serious environmental threat to good health for developed countries. Many believe the curse of industrial society lies in the ill health caused by such pollutants. No data exist on the direct relationship between pollution and ill health, but toxic disposal sites such as Love Canal, New York, or Times Beach, Missouri have convinced the world of a direct correlation. Cancer, which may be a direct result of toxic pollution, will likely strike one out of every four Americans. It is already the primary cause of death for children.

The US Environmental Protection Agency has estimated that more than 250 million tons of hazardous materials are added to the environment each year. This amounts to one ton of such waste per person. Most of this material will lead to irreversible contamination and while contamination touches all of our lives, actually, like many social evils, the disposal of hazardous materials has serious racial and economic overtones. Communities without strong leadership or strong legislative representation tend to become the sites for dumps and disposal facilities. One thinks particularly of Indian reservations where people already shamefully treated are suffering even more injustices due to toxic waste dumping. In most of the communities where landfills were placed blacks make up the majority of the population.

Given the severity of the problem the faith community could take the following actions:

—inform all its members about the health hazards of pollutants;

—lobby for stronger legislation in the disposal of hazardous materials;

—encourage technological study which might lead to safer disposal methods;

—cooperate with minorities to develop stronger political leadership;

—take leadership roles in waste management projects in order to develop mutually acceptable disposal systems;

—work with business and industry to seek wholistic health as well as economic health for a community.

The Judeo-Christian faith community has passed through the theological problem of universal self-destruction. The story of the flood and Noah is intended to teach us a key point in our faith: human unfaithfulness can lead to world destruction. The rainbow symbolizes a rejection of that possibility. God (the beginning and end of this world) and humanity are wedded infinitely. As children of God we stand against those forces which would "flood" the world with destruction. As children of God we also work together with those forces which will reunite creator and creation in a healthy and safe environment.

In light of the crises which face us all, many have proposed the adoption of the Shakertown Pledge for every Christian. From a believers' church perspective, this is an excellent idea.

Recognizing that the earth and the fullness thereof is a gift from our gracious God, and that we are called to cherish, nurture, and provide loving stewardship for the earth's resources;

And recognizing that life itself is a gift, and a call to responsibility, joy, and celebration;

I make the following declarations:

1. *I declare myself to be a world citizen.*
2. *I commit myself to lead an ecologically sound life.*
3. *I commit myself to lead a life of creative simplicity and to share my personal wealth with the world's poor.*
4. *I commit myself to join with others in reshaping institutions in order to bring about a more just global society in which each person has full access to the needed resources for their physical, emotional, intellectual, and spiritual growth.*
5. *I commit myself to occupational accountability, and in so doing I will seek to avoid the creation of products which cause harm to others.*

6. *I affirm the gift of my body, and commit myself to its proper nourishment and physical well-being.*

7. *I commit myself to examine continually my relations with others, and to attempt to relate honestly, morally, and lovingly to those around me.*

8. *I commit myself to personal renewal through prayer, meditation, and study.*

9. *I commit myself to responsible participation in a community of faith.*

Case Study

The area called the Horn of Africa (especially Ethiopia and Sudan) has historically suffered severe droughts. For the last twenty years the drought and subsequent famine has been especially severe. The last catastrophic famine occurred in 1973–74. In the winter of 1984–85 another diasater occurred. About Christmastime an estimated 7,750,000 were threatened with starvation. Approximately 6,400 died each day. Various agencies responded with assistance. The United States government pledged 50,000 tons of grain from its stockpiled surpluses. Many felt that was not enough. The lobbying group Bread for the World sought a much larger grant. Senator Paul Simon introduced measures that would spend a billion dollars for relief. His brother, Arthur Simon, head of Bread for the World, tried to assist. It was very difficult to move the government because Ethiopia, the hardest hit by famine, was anti-American. Ethiopia hardly acknowledged the American help and the USSR, Ethiopia's supporter, pledged 10,000 tons of grain.

Meanwhile, private relief agencies were more successful. A variety of agencies promised 550,000 tons and made an agreement with the Ethiopian government for distribution. Many argued that private organizations could not effect a just distribution of the grain. Some agencies, already working in the Horn area, continued to pursue the development of agriculture (especially irrigation) for the stricken region.

Questions for Discussion:

1. The Horn of Africa is known to be stricken with famine. What is the responsibility of the community of nations toward such a region? Does that responsibility occur only at times of catastrophes?

2. Given the resources in the world, are some states not economically viable? Which ones should not be encouraged?

3. Should Christians press more for governmental relief action or give aid through church agencies? If you think you should support church agencies, to which ones would you, or do you, send money?

11

Genetic Engineering

While the issue of genetic engineering is being discussed today as if it were something new, that is not really the case. Western civilization has partially depended on the skills of persons to breed certain plants and animals in such a way that the new plants or animals would benefit humanity. The characteristics of all living things depend on genes carried by the "eggs and sperms" of plants and animals. Certain genes can be encouraged to be dominant while others can be encouraged to be recessive. This genetic process is called selective breeding and the domestication of certain animals has depended on it. The development of more useful and better agricultural products has depended on genetic engineering as well. Most of us happily make use of the results of such experiments.

In 1944 the science of genetics took a new turn. The chemical nature of hereditary material was discovered. This material, Deoxyribonucleic Acid (known as DNA), was the object of considerable research. In 1953 James Watson and Francis Crick discovered the chemical structure of the material. At that point biochemists and molecular biologists gained access to the genes themselves. They could create DNA in their own laboratories. The goal for many scientists has been to locate and gain access to all of the genes (about

50,000). By 1986 some 800 gene locations had been identified and isolated. With even this much information certain
gains in health care can be realized. The potential for the
future seems staggering. There are 4,000 known genetic diseases, including cystic fibrosis, hemophilia, Huntington's
Disease, and muscular dystrophy, to mention a few of the
more well-known. About 1.2 million people are hospitalized
annually because of genetic "diseases" (disorders). Genetic
diseases cause a fifth of all infant deaths and are responsible
for forty percent of pediatric admissions to health care
facilities and thirteen percent of adult admissions.

Plants

There are various possibilities for genetic engineering. Among
the most promising are advances in the field of horticulture.
Just as agriculturalists and scientists have already worked to
produce better agricultural plants and stock animals, and their
by-products, so genetic engineering simply multiplies the
possibilities. In some cases it will be possible to increase the
nutritional value of grains and vegetables by increasing the
quantity and/or quality of the protein content, for example, by
increasing the solid content of a tomato. In other cases plants
can be created which are resistant to drought or excessive salt.
Perhaps most widely discussed at the moment is the possibility
of extending the freezeline for agriculture by developing plants
which can withstand a few degrees more cold. Or, in another
direction, scientists can create hybrids of two different plants by
means of what is called protoplast fusion. An example would
be a pomato which grows potatoes underground and
tomatoes above the ground.

In terms of world hunger the positive aspects cannot be
overestimated. Plants can be produced which will grow better
in environments now unproductive, and the nutritional
quality of the products can be increased. Even without
specific results of genetic engineering, countries like Israel

and Iceland have demonstrated what can be done with what was considered environments alien to agriculture.

Opposition to such research does come from some environmentalists such as Jeremy Rifkin. While they do not object to the anticipated gains, they fear that the very research itself, or even the new plants, could release side-effects which would be detrimental to both humans and nature. Stated in "beneficence" terms discussed earlier the harm could outweigh the gains. It is difficult to evaluate these arguments, since the potential side-effects are unknown. By and large Christians, with permission to have dominion (Genesis 1), have not hesitated to "improve creation." To most it would seem that the possibility of a greatly increased food production would be a gain we dare not refuse.

Animals

Presumably the same type of gains in animal husbandry could be achieved as in plant genetic engineering. At this time there are no such examples, yet one can imagine leaner, more nutritious cuts of meat. One of the major ethical issues, however, is the patenting of "new animals." Some Christian groups oppose this possibility. In contrast to plant genetics this appears to be a more serious threat to human life. The alteration of human types, it is argued, would be only a step away. On the other hand, it seems to many other Christians that the world would gain by the creation of cows which could give greater milk production in less developed areas of the world. Nevertheless, experimentation with animals for mere curiosity is clearly more culpable than experimentation with plants. Christians will oppose the destruction of animals without good cause as well as the creation of mutants, sports, and genetic mavericks.

Pharmaceuticals

Since genes can be synthesized, it is now possible to let them work for us as if they were in the human body. It has become possible to produce industrially what otherwise had to come from human or animal sources. Most notable is the production of insulin for diabetics. By placing the gene coded for insulin in an appropriate environment, human insulin can be grown. Heretofore it was necessary to use animal-derived insulin. The gain for health care can hardly be imagined. It is possible that the greatest gain for molecular biology in health care will prove to be in the field of pharmaceuticals. Several new drugs of the interferon type may have an affect against cancer cells. A blood factor known as VIII aids hemophiliacs by clotting the blood. The list grows daily.

Granted the risks of synthetic gene research, it seems to most Christians that these breakthroughs are a cause for rejoicing. Many persons whose lives were foreshortened or severely limited can now enjoy life to a fuller extent.

Humans

We have already suggested some benefits for health care which might result from genetic engineering. The potential harm is also greater at the human level, of course. In the hands of some military or racist groups, uses of genetic engineering might move society closer to forms of slavery even more devastating than the nuclear bomb. It is too soon to comment on the types of biological weapons that might be developed. Surely any medical technology that can change health and personality for the good can be used for evil intent as well.

For those in the Free Church tradition, the theological issues are as revolutionary as scientific ones. Most opponents of genetic engineering are disturbed by any tampering with God's creation. That argument probably cannot be sustained. As has been mentioned throughout this chapter, a part of "civilizing" is to alter the natural ordered functions of plants and animals. Agriculturalists have done that for centuries. To avoid tampering with creation, there would have to be an international return to nature. Some in the believers' churches have opted for nature as seen in Thoreau's Walden or in the communal society of a Bruderhof or Ephrata Cloister. But the majority have bypassed that solution. Furthermore, theologically speaking, we cannot return to the Garden of Eden—pristine Paradise. We are kept from the Garden by our sin—the alienation created in our formation. The issue is not a return, but a future.

Because the Christian tradition considers distrust, or lack of faith, as the cause for our alienation from God and the world, it stands to reason that the end time will be a moment of reconciliation and restored trust. The believers' churches are torn both ways. They often look back to the "golden age" of the New Testament, or perhaps to their denominational origins. Yet we also look forward to the New Jerusalem and so live and work in order to make such a time possible.

The theological issue facing us has to do with the basic definition of end time. Is it not necessary for the end time to be a time of human and divine trust? Is that not a religious, psychological, and sociological reality? Can it ever be achieved by scientific means? To put it more directly: can those of us who pray and work for peace ever be satisfied with a forced or artificial peace? If we could hypnotize all the generals in the world and order them to think only of peace, would we be satisfied? Presumably not. Peace will not occur until people live justly with each other and treat each other as peers of the coming kingdom. A forced answer must be defined as an undesirable answer.

Genetic engineering promises to give us a better life. It also promises to eradicate some health problems which are associated with evils that modern, industrial society has developed, for example, cancer. Shall we promote the cure or shall we insist on attacking the cause? The approach I have taken throughout this discussion is that Christians would be well advised to *allow* the cure but *to work simultaneously on the causes*. Genetic engineering will be a useful tool for good health only when we constantly seek to change a society that causes ill health.

For the most part national judicatories and the scientific community will need to keep church bodies informed about genetic engineering. This technology will affect each person, but decision making will be more of an issue with the faith community and larger society than a private concern. Above all, Christians need to work for appropriate social guidelines, be aware of the dangers that might develop, and know the positive possibilities that will surely touch us all.

Case Study

A forty-seven-year-old engineer has polycystic kidney disease, in his case a genetic disorder, and must have his blood purified by hemodialysis with an artificial kidney machine. Victims of the disease usually die a few years after symptoms appear, often in their forties, though dialysis and transplants can be life-saving for several years. The patient has two children: a son, eighteen, just starting college, and a daughter, sixteen. Though the parents know that the disease is genetic—that their children may carry it and might transmit it to their offspring—the son and daughter are not told about the nature of the genetic disorder. The parents insist the children should not be told because it would frighten them unnecessarily, inhibit their social life, and make them feel hopeless about the future. They are firm in saying that the hospital staff should not tell the children. The knowledge, they believe, is privileged and must be kept secret. Yet the hospital staff are concerned about the children innocently involving their future spouses and victimizing their own children. (Taken from *Hard Choices*, p. 9)

Questions for Discussion:

1. Given the present state of genetic research, under what circumstances, if any, should genetic information ever be withheld from your children?

2. What responsibility do the health care personnel have to the parents? To the children?

3. In what sense is withholding information a form of "false witness"? What damage could it do in this case?

12

Congregational Strategies in Health Care

This chapter suggests some ways in which the local congregation can aid its members and its neighborhood in the process of making health care decisions and improving health for people in our time and for future generations.

Congregational Health Care Committees

The issues surrounding health care have become so complex that individual decision making is often ill advised and unnecessarily self-oriented. Most persons do consult with friends and health experts before making a decision. A growing number of church leaders are advocating that the faith community should develop health care committees or task forces which could serve as advisory groups, support networks, and conveyors of information. Such groups might be composed of at least one health care professional, a person interested in ethics, a person who networks well with the congregation and the community, a "patient," and a person who can work with local hospitals or health care institutions. The committee would serve primarily as a team which could give support to members of the faith community facing health care decisions. If desired, the same group would also be prepared to share whatever information and advice which might be useful. Unless the local church could utilize more than one committee, the same group should keep the congregation apprised of recent health care developments, current legislative and legal issues, and important public debates about health care ethics. For some congregations in the believers' church tradition, the health care committee would simply be an extension of the duties exercised by deacons. Deacons would normally set up care for those who need assistance as well as visit the sick (see 1 Timothy 3:8–13).

While these committees or task forces are to serve primarily the congregation and the local community, two important connections should be maintained: one with local hospitals and health care institutions, and a second with denominational boards and agencies.

Hospital and Institutional Ethics Committees

Many health care institutions have established ethics committees. Many mainline and Free Church denominations are calling for such committees and the President's Commission for the Study of Ethical Problems in Medicine recommends that health care institutions establish ethics committees. Some states are even considering making such committees mandatory. These committees have at least four functions.

1. Prognosis

The public pressure for ethics committees arises from the Karen Quinlan case. In 1975 the Supreme Court of New Jersey ruled that if the guardian and/or family of Karen Quinlan wished to withdraw life support no physician or medical body could prevent that. The court ruled that the family's wishes could be carried out *if* the hospital ethics committee, or a like body, concurred. In other words, if the ethics committee agreed that Karen's case was hopeless, then life supports could be withdrawn. Karen was in a coma and the support system was withdrawn without her consent.

This action set the legal pattern for a controversial function of ethics committees. In the Quinlan case, the decision was not binding; still their recommendations could be used as a means of gaining implied consent. If ethics committees have a prognosis function, then either health care and legal experts must be appointed to the committee or be available for consultation.

2. Review ethical decisions for individual patients

Much like the committee that operates within the faith community, the institutional committee should assist patients, their families, and the hospital in making good decisions about patient care. Obviously, this function deals with many of the issues that have been raised in this study. Should a physician be allowed to do a bone marrow transplant on a patient who has other terminal problems? When should extraordinary means be used? Of course, the advice of such committees cannot be mandated.

3. Make larger ethical and policy decisions

These decisions deal primarily with justice issues. The institutional ethics committee would recommend methods, if not solutions, for the use of scarce resources. For example, how would the hospital decide between two children who need a liver transplant when there is only one donor organ available? Again, the function of the committee is advisory, but if it represents sufficient concerns it can be considered the best advice available.

4. Counseling

Finally the ethics committee could give counsel to both patient and health care professional. Normally, counseling would come from other sources such as pastors and medical social workers, but there may be a conflict, occasionally, which could best be handled by the hospital committee.

Such a committee almost always has on it a physician and a minister or chaplain. Many also have a nurse and a hospital administrator. Others include an attorney, a medical social worker, a representative from the community, and sometimes patients. Access to the committee represents a particular difficulty. In most cases only the physicians and hospital administration bring agenda to the committee. It is considered inappropriate by some for patients to know of a committee that could make recommendations regarding their health care. Such confidentiality, however, prevents patients from bringing their agenda to the table. Mutuality would dictate that the hospital ethics committee be a known entity available through the office of admissions as well as the chaplain.

Denominational Boards and Agencies

Many denominations, large and small, have created regional or national health and welfare committees. These committees typically listen to concerns of the local congregations and channel them to larger national issues. They also provide education and identify concerns for denominational advocacy. In this way the ethics committee of the local congregation can be informed about national and international health problems. Regional health and welfare committees should not only include representatives from the local congregations, but also regional task forces and advocacy groups. Among these should be task groups representing concerns of older adults, substance abuse, handicapped, mental health, children, family abuse, and wholistic health.

Wholistic Health

Since 1970 several local congregations in the United States have sponsored wholistic health centers. These centers are more complex than ethics committees and not every congregation could or should enter this realm. The movement for wholistic health centers was founded by Granger Westberg, a Lutheran minister and educator, out of the conviction that wellness has as much to do with faith as it does with medicine. Wholistic health centers, as they have now developed, include space for ministers, counselors, and physicians. Diagnosis is done in terms of a client's faith, personal well-being, and physical condition. In addition to the community service performed by wholistic health centers, it can be extremely beneficial for the church as well. Cooperating with the congregational health care committee, the center can establish classes in wellness such as aerobics and dieting. A number of churches also now have self-help groups akin to Alcoholics Anonymous that deal with overweight, abuse, sex, and chemical dependency.

Church Nurse Program

A variation of the wholistic health center, also proposed by Granger Westberg, is the presence of a church nurse on the staff of the local congregation. The nurse can relate to the health problems of the congregation in the context of faith. At the same time a nurse can relate helpfully to the congregational health care committee and the hospital committee on ethics. The church nurse can carry out certain health care functions, such as advising, taking blood checks, giving counsel on diets and preventive medicine. The nurse can also become an advocate for programs, such as Medicaid and Medicare, so that persons can receive the best health care available. In some instances a congregation can work with a hospice to develop a nursing program, though then the nurse's function will center on aging and dying. In any case most church nurse programs have started when the local church purchased shared time from a local health care institution.

Hospices

As indicated in the section on the end of life, life is understood to consist of the network of interrelationships which compose our social being. Death can be defined, therefore, as the cessation of those networks. People who are terminally ill ought to be allowed to die in circumstances where relationships can be enhanced. Isolation at such a time comes close to sin itself. In the past almost no hospitals made arrangements for the "communal" or networking death of a patient. The private sector, as well as some hospitals, now has begun to develop hospices for the terminally ill. It is the opinion of many that every local congregation should have a liaison with, and support, a hospice. In this way members of the congregation have access to a place where death can occur with dignity and in a faith context.

Case Study

In 1954 Mary Anne Monahan was born in a hospital for unwed mothers. Four weeks later she was adopted by Joseph and Julia Quinlan of Roxbury Township, New Jersey. Named Karen by her adoptive parents, she was raised in a Roman Catholic context. Karen's childhood was uneventful, but in 1975 Karen's behavior began to change. On the night of April 14 she apparently swallowed some tranquilizers and then drank several gin-and-tonics with her friends. She fell unconscious. Though she was treated immediately, she never regained consciousness.

After three months in a coma, her parents asked her doctors to take Karen off life-support systems. The doctors refused. The parents went to court to ask permission for Karen to die with dignity. Such permission had never been granted before. The lawyer for the Quinlans argued it was inhumane to keep her alive, while the lawyer for the doctors argued the state could not be sure of Karen's prognosis. The judge ruled for the doctors.

The Quinlans appealed to the New Jersey Supreme Court. On March 31, 1976, the court ruled that if the family of Karen and the attending physicians agreed there was no reasonable possibility for recovery, then they should consult with an ethics committee of the hospital. If that body agreed then the present life-support system could be withdrawn.

The support system (respirator) was withdrawn. Karen lived until June of 1985.

Questions for Discussion:

1. Who, if anyone, besides Karen herself had the right to consent to the removal of life-support systems?

2. Under what circumstances would you allow a hospital ethics committee to determine whether you should continue with a life-support system?

3. Would you serve on a church committee which had the power to give advice regarding life, death, and major medical procedures? If not you, then who should serve on such a committee?

Conclusion

It would be presumptuous to make excessive claims for any attempt to apply a particular theological tradition to a controversial and complex field such as health care ethics. This work is no exception. Yet tolerant humility does not seem appropriate either. The notion of covenant is not just another idea or another tradition. It lies at the heart of the biblical faith. It is also not appropriate to suppose the ethic described here applies only to those who adhere to believers' church tradition.

The voluntary, believers' church cannot be relegated to the sideshow of religious history. Loosely defined, there are today more believers' churches than any other type. Some historians have observed that all churches in America have become voluntary. There is no legally favored church; all must compete for members and financial resources. If that observation is true, almost every tradition—Protestant and Catholic—must deal with a faith community of adults who support the church for reasons rooted in voluntarism. In other countries the revolutions of communism and secularism have also forced state-supported churches into a period of disestablishment. The churches of China, Russia, and Western Europe are beginning to look very much like the faith community described in these pages.

A church that no longer can assume national support or loyalty of the ruling classes will need to relate to public policy without public power. The ethic described in this book seeks to gain adherents by an expression of community self-understanding and not by accepted public norms. The voluntary church today does not control those forces which can enforce a public ethical norm.

Even more than the disestablishment of mainline churches and the deconstruction of a public Christian ethical stance, the bankruptcy of western individualism calls believers to an ethic based on community relationships instead of personal choice and freedom. Persons are formed in a social context and they live in a continuing community. Decisions are made on the basis of formations and the most valuable relationships. The Christian faith cannot ultimately depend on personal conversions, rational arguments, or even divine obligations. The vitality of the Christian faith depends on the social context in which people live, the formation which creates them as persons, and the faith stories that inform their decisions.

In that sense the ethical stance taken in this study is not an option. To be sure, some of the applications suggested may be inappropriate, but the presuppositions cannot easily be set aside. It is my hope this book will enable congregations to face tough choices with a feeling of hope, a sense of direction, and the certainty that decisions made within the faith community have ultimate significance.

Resources for Further Study

Beauchamp, Tom L. and Childress, James F. *Principles of Biomedical Ethics*. 2nd edition. Oxford: Oxford University Press, 1983. The basic textbook on health care ethics.

Biomedical-Ethical Issues, ed. by Frank M. Harron. New Haven, CT: Yale University Press, 1983. A source book of legal statements and policy statements.

Childress, James F., *Priorities in Biomedical Ethics*. Philadelphia: Westminster, 1981. A volume that discusses issues such as research and technology, in addition to the topics covered in this study.

Congregational Wellness Manual. Goshen, IN: Mennonite Mutual Aid, 1983. An excellent program and manual for health care in a local congregation.

DuFresne, Florine. *Home Care: An Alternative to the Nursing Home*. Elgin, IL: Brethren Press, 1984. A how-to book on the hospice-type care at home.

The Encyclopedia of Bioethics, ed. by W. T. Reich. New York: Free Press, 1978. A standard reference.

Gustafson, James M., *Ethics from a Theocentric Perspective,* 2 vols. Chicago: University of Chicago Press 1981, 1984. The secoond volume deals with assumptions of philosophical and Christian ethics in considerable depth. The sections on suicide and world hunger are very helpful.

Hard Choices. Department of Education, KCTS/Seattle. The text of an excellent television series on medical ethics.

Harron, Frank, John Burnside, and Tom Beauchamp. *Health and Human Values.* New Haven, CT: Yale University Press, 1983. A solid discussion of the same issues treated in this volume.

Hastings Center Studies. Briarcliff Manor, New York. The primary source for the most recent materials on health care ethics.

Hauerwas, Stanley. *A Community of Character.* Notre Dame, IN: University of Notre Dame, 1981. A significant series of essays in which the author develops a virtue or character ethic from a Free Church position.
_____. *Suffering Presence.* Notre Dame, IN: University of Notre Dame, 1986. A well known Free Church ethicist applies his position to issues involving medicine, and the mentally handicapped.

Jury, Mark and Dan Jury. *Gramp.* New York: Grossman, 1976. A personal account about care for the elderly.

MacIntyre, Alasdair. *After Virtue,* 2nd ed. Notre Dame, IN: University of Notre Dame, 1984. The primary philosophical discussion of virtue ethics.

McClendon, James Wm. *Ethics.* Nashville: Abingdon, 1986. A work on theological ethics written by a Free Church scholar who utilizes the narrative approach.

Medical Ethics, Human Choices. A Christian Perspective, John Rogers, ed., Scottdale, PA: Herald Press, 1988. Several religious and medical professionals address issues in health care from a believers' church perspective.

Miller-McLemore, Bonnie. *Death, Sin and the Moral Life.* Decatur, GA: Scholar's Press, 1988. A theological perspective on health care ethics.

Nelson, J. Robert. *Human Life.* Philadelphia: Fortress, 1984. A basic book about life decisions, including medical decisions. Based on biblical insights.

Rhoads, David and Donald Michie. *Mark as Story.* Philadelphia: Fortress, 1982. An excellent study of the narrative form of a Gospel.

Stoddard, Sandol. *The Hospice Movement.* New York: Stein and Day, 1978. A frequently used introduction to hospice care.

Totan, Suzanne C. *World Hunger.* Maryknoll, NY: Orbis, 1982. Discusses the reasons for hunger, the facts about world and hunger, and suggests some actions to be taken.

Varga, Andrew C. *The Main Issues in Bioethics.* New York: Paulist Press, 1984. A key textbook on medical ethics.

Via, Dan O.,Jr., *The Ethics of Mark's Gospel in the Middle of Time.* Philadelphia: Fortress, 1985. A unique study of Mark's gospel from the perspective of narrative ethics.

Westberg, Granger E., ed. *Theological Roots of Wholistic Health.* Hinsdale, IL: Wholistic Health Centers, 1979. A book on the reason for and establishment of wholistic health centers, edited by the "father" of congregational health care programs.